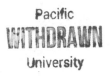
TAKE CONTROL OF YOUR DRINKING
. . . AND YOU MAY NOT NEED TO QUIT

TAKE

Control

OF YOUR

Drinking

...And You
May Not Need
to Quit

MICHAEL S. LEVY, PH.D.

THE JOHNS HOPKINS UNIVERSITY PRESS

BALTIMORE

© 2007 Michael S. Levy

All rights reserved. Published 2007

Printed in the United States of America on acid-free paper

9 8 7 6 5 4 3 2 1

The Johns Hopkins University Press
2715 North Charles Street
Baltimore, Maryland 21218-4363
www.press.jhu.edu

Library of Congress Cataloging-in-Publication Data

Levy, Michael S., 1953–

    Take control of your drinking—and you may not need to
quit / Michael S. Levy.

      p. cm.

    Includes bibliographical references and index.

    ISBN-13: 978-0-8018-8667-6 (hardcover : alk. paper)

    ISBN-13: 978-0-8018-8668-3 (pbk. : alk. paper)

    ISBN-10: 0-8018-8667-8 (hardcover : alk. paper)

    ISBN-10: 0-8018-8668-6 (pbk. : alk. paper)

    1. Drinking of alcoholic beverages. 2. Temperance.

3. Alcoholism—Treatment. I. Title.

HV5035.L48 2007

613.81—dc22   2006101452

A catalog record for this book is available from
the British Library.

*Special discounts are available for bulk purchases
of this book. For more information, please contact
Special Sales at 410-516-6936 or specialsales@press.jhu.edu.*

CONTENTS

PART V ■ OTHER RESOURCES

INTRODUCTION

I STARTED WORKING with people who were hurting themselves by drinking too much about 20 years ago. At that time, the three most important principles I was taught were: (1) people *had* to admit that they had the disease of *alcoholism*; (2) people *had* to stop drinking entirely; and (3) people *had* to get treatment if they were going to stop alcohol from ruining their lives. And treatment in most every case meant going to Alcoholics Anonymous (AA) meetings, because AA was the only approach believed to work. If people wouldn't admit they had a disease, or they refused to stop drinking, or they simply wouldn't go to AA meetings, this was a sign of their *denial,* or their unwillingness to admit they had a drinking problem.

In fact, the AA expression, "Keep it simple, stupid," applied not only to the alcoholic but also to the professional who was treating the person. Don't do anything fancy or different—just get the alcoholic to admit that he or she is an alcoholic, get the person to stop drinking, and get the person to go to "90 meetings in 90 days."

I was even told that I shouldn't treat alcoholics in psychotherapy. Exploring how drinking may have something to do with patients' emotional life was in contrast to the idea that their problem with alcohol was a primary disease that had nothing to do with anything else, especially their psychological lives. The message I received was that seeing alcoholics in therapy instead of insisting they go to AA meetings would simply increase their denial and foster the idea that they didn't have a disease.

Unfortunately, I found that many people resisted one or more of these well-intended suggestions. Some reported that they had checked out the AA scene, but it just wasn't for them. They told me that instead of going to meetings, they preferred to spend their time doing something more fun than listening to alcoholics talk about their problems. Some even said that they hated AA meetings. Reasons included not liking the spiritual overtones in AA meetings and not liking the rigid approach that can be suggested in AA. Others seemed to be private people who didn't like the public exposure of going to meetings. And others even told me that going to meetings made them want to drink more! Rather than hearing all of the talk about drinking and the problems drinking caused, these people wanted to put their alcohol problems behind them and not be constantly reminded of them.

What was most interesting to me was that many of these people admitted that they had an alcohol problem, and it didn't seem like they were *in denial.* They just didn't like going to meetings. These people preferred working with a therapist on an individual basis. What was I to do? Refuse to see them, or work with them in the manner they wanted? And what if I continued to see them and they continued to drink? Was I doing them a disservice by seeing them in therapy? Was I making things worse and giving them the wrong care?

There were some people who refused to admit that they had the disease of *alcoholism.* They told me that they didn't like being labeled an *alcoholic.* This label made them feel as if something was terribly wrong with them. On the other hand, they could admit that they had a drinking problem, and they acknowledged that they often drank too much. Some viewed their problem with alcohol simply as a bad habit that they had learned over time.

In my opinion, many of these people weren't in denial. While refusing to acknowledge the idea that they were alcoholic was for some a way to minimize their problem, for others this was not true. Many knew that they had to do something about their drinking and that drinking was clearly a problem for them. They just didn't like being labeled alcoholic. This forced me to question how important it was for people with a drinking problem to admit they had the disease of alcoholism. Wasn't it fine for people to view their alcohol problem however they wished? Wasn't it more important for people to develop a plan to address their drinking rather than to get them to believe a particular concept? Who cares what they call their problem? More important is that they do something about it.

I worked with some people who wanted to try to moderate or control their drinking instead of choosing to become abstinent. I was totally unprepared for this, as everything I had learned told me that people needed to stop drinking completely in order to get better. In fact, I had learned that the wish to moderate drinking was the most blatant form of denial, as it represented a refusal to acknowledge powerlessness over alcohol consumption. The whole nature of *alcoholism* is that people cannot moderate their drinking and must become abstinent to get better. Trying to control drinking was a clear sign: these people were not admitting they had a drinking problem, and they were still in denial.

What was I to do in this circumstance? Confront them about their denial and their unwillingness to do what it takes to get better? Should I tell them that their wish to try to moderate their drinking is just that—a wish—and that trying to control problem drinking simply isn't possible? I certainly didn't want to do anything that would further their denial. Or should I work with them in their goal to try to moderate their drinking? Maybe I needed to do this as a way to engage them into the treatment process. Even if it wasn't possible to control their drinking, perhaps they needed to go through this process so they could figure out that moderating drinking *wasn't* possible for them.

I was in a quandary. First, I was concerned that I'd be viewed as a quack if I worked with people to help them to moderate their drinking. I might be laughed at, and my stature as a psychologist who knew something about alcohol problems might be diminished. I was also concerned about my professional liability if people didn't get better and drinking continued to cause them harm. Maybe I would be held legally liable if people's continued drinking hurt them.

At the same time, I was beginning to see that the "one size fits all" approach simply didn't work, and that if I was going to be successful, people needed to be given the freedom to make their own decisions. If people first wanted to try to moderate their drinking, perhaps they should be given this choice. And again, maybe they needed to discover whether controlling their drinking was possible before they would consider abstaining from alcohol completely.

Fortunately, I had some supervisors who had a flexible approach and gave me the freedom and permission to work with people in less traditional ways. I am reminded of a conversation I had with one of my supervisors early on in my training. I told him that I was seeing some people with alcohol problems in my private practice who continued to drink and who refused to admit that they were alcoholic. They also refused to make full use of AA meetings in the community. I wondered whether I should continue to see them or whether I should terminate therapy, as they weren't entirely ready for treatment. My inclination was to continue to work with them, but I questioned that stance based upon what I had learned. What my supervisor said to me was that I would have an extremely small practice if I only saw people who admitted they were alcoholics, who went to AA meetings consistently, and who never drank. I would also be limiting myself to only the easiest of patients.

I was discovering that different things worked with different people and that individuals *must be allowed to find out for themselves what they need to do to get their lives in order.* I knew this from my general clinical training, and I simply started to apply this thinking to the treatment of people who struggled with alcohol. As straightforward as this idea may seem, it was revolutionary at the time.

As my confidence grew and I gained more experience in the treatment of drinking problems, I began to see that no two people who struggled with alcohol consumption were the same. While some had very serious problems with alcohol and clearly needed to stop drinking to avoid destroying their lives, others seemed to get by for years, though they drank problematically, and their lives didn't seem to get worse and worse and worse. Others had a pattern of not drinking for long periods of time, interspersed with brief periods of heavy drinking. I also saw some adolescents and young adults who struggled with alcohol but who seemed to mature out of their difficulties essentially on their own.

And my instinct that different approaches worked with different people was confirmed. For some, AA was a godsend; for others, it provided no benefit. And some people obtained help from other types of self-help meetings. For many people, abstinence was the only route to recovery; others learned to drink less and moderate their drinking. I also discovered that many people stopped alcohol from ruining their lives without outside help of any kind, or through an extremely limited contact with treatment. They just seemed to make up their mind to change their lives and their relationship to alcohol.

I also got the opportunity to meet some people who had been in and out of the treatment system for years due to heavy drinking and seemed as if they would never stop drinking and get their lives together. Then at some point, something seemed to click, and they were able to stop drinking. Treatment appeared to be almost the *least* important factor in this; what seemed most important was their *internal motivation and desire to change.*

All of these observations surprised me, because I had been taught that treatment was essential and that if left untreated, alcoholism was a chronic, progressive, and fatal disease. I had learned that the phrase "the man takes a drink, the drink takes a drink, and the drink takes the man" applied to everyone. In order to avoid a mental hospital, jail, or death, a person diagnosed with alcoholism had no choice but to get treatment and to stop drinking entirely. I came to realize that this was not entirely true.

▢ ▢ ▢

After working in this field for many years and refining how I worked with people, I decided to write a book for people who struggle in some way with alcohol. In this book I would summarize my thinking about alcohol problems and my treatment approach. I decided to do this for three main reasons. First, there is considerable misunderstanding about the nature and treatment of alcohol problems that I want to dispel. Having an alcohol problem is now an "out of the closet" subject, and many people know something about this topic. As the saying goes, "a little knowledge is dangerous," and I want to give people *more* knowledge so that they are better informed. People who are affected by an alcohol problem and those who love them should have this knowledge and should not be misinformed.

Second, I wanted to write a book that offers people an approach they can use to *help themselves* with a drinking problem regardless of how they choose to understand or address it. In fact, I wanted to write a book that gives people total control and complete freedom over how they choose to perceive and address their problem. People should not be forced to believe a certain idea or be told what to do to resolve a drinking problem. They should be free to understand their problem with alcohol in any way they want. They should also be free to discover what they need to do in order to stop alcohol from ruining their lives.

Finally, it became obvious to me that many, many people do not seek and do not want to seek treatment for their alcohol problem. There are many reasons why people do not get outside help. They may be too ashamed or embarrassed to ask for help, or they may simply be private people who do not like sharing the intimate aspects of their lives with strangers. Some people prefer to do things on their own and don't like having to rely on others. And some, while concerned about their drinking, believe that going to treatment means that they will have to stop drinking, which they are not ready to do. Providing a resource that allows people to help themselves on their own was another reason I wrote this book.

HOW TO TELL IF YOU NEED THIS BOOK

According to the National Institute on Alcohol Abuse and Alcoholism (NIAAA), approximately 18 million adults in the United States either abuse or are dependent upon alcohol. And for each of these individuals, there are many others who are at risk for severe consequences related to drinking. These are problem drinkers who don't quite meet the criteria for alcohol abuse or dependence but who sometimes or frequently exceed moderate drinking levels.

Many of these people know and admit that they have an alcohol problem, yet they simply do not want to see a therapist. Nor do they want to attend Alcoholics Anonymous or other self-help meetings. Whether it is the stigma of having an alcohol problem, not knowing who to turn to, or the cost of treatment, they do not get the help they need. If you are among the individuals in this group, this book is for you. It will help you to help yourself with your drinking in the privacy of your own home.

Other people are not sure if they have a problem with alcohol consumption. While they have noticed patterns of drinking that worry them, they do not know whether alcohol is truly a problem for them. They are not ready or willing to enter the treatment world or self-help world. If you are among those individuals, this book also is for you. It will help you to decide whether you have a drinking problem and, if you do, what you can do about it.

Perhaps you see yourself as having a drinking problem and have seen a therapist, but your treatment did not go well. Or perhaps you attended AA or other self-help meetings, but those did not go well either. You may feel discouraged and may have given up on yourself. Whatever problems you may have had with drinking and whatever treatment you may have had, this book is for you. It will help you to answer the following questions:

Do You Have an Alcohol Problem?

Chapter 1 will help you to make a realistic appraisal of whether you have a drinking problem, and if so, the extent of it. You will be asked to reflect in detail on your past drinking and any difficulties you have experienced that were in any way related to your use of alcohol. You will also begin to evaluate the damage your alcohol consumption may have done to yourself and to your relationships. By the end of this chapter you will know whether your use of alcohol is problematic and whether you need to change your pattern of drinking.

If You Have an Alcohol Problem, Why Is This So?

Many individuals who have a problem with alcohol consumption wonder why they do. The next chapter reviews the prevailing ideas and explanations for some people's difficulty with controlling their alcohol intake. The goal is to help you to understand why you may have a drinking problem and to ensure that you will not beat yourself up for a having a problem with alcohol.

Where to Begin?

Many people recognize that they have an alcohol problem but just don't know where to start. For example, how to get and stay motivated is a frequent question. In fact, having some mixed feelings about changing is very common. A part of you may want to change, but there is another part that wants to keep things the way they have always been. It is also easy for motivation to slip after you get started. Chapter 3 will help you to understand why this happens and how to stay on course.

People also often wonder whether it is possible for them to help themselves or whether they need to get treatment. The truth is that many people have been able to help themselves without outside assistance of any kind. Research has shown that about 75 percent of people with alcohol-related problems who recover do so without any formal help. In fact, not only is it possible for you to help yourself with your drinking problem, but you *must* help yourself. Whether you seek help from others or try to stop or moderate your drinking on your own, success will rest primarily with you.

Chapter 4 explodes the myth that treatment is essential and shows that many people with drinking problems are able to help themselves. More important, it outlines the mental state that you will need to have if you are going to be successful. Chapter 5 will help you decide whether you will need medical assistance to safely eliminate alcohol from your body. Whatever course you take, freeing yourself from the toxicity of alcohol will be crucial to your success.

Another question is whether completely stopping alcohol must be the way to go, or whether you could try to moderate their drinking by learning to drink less. Chapter 6 will review this question and help you to decide how you should proceed.

ABSTINENCE OR MODERATION?

This book offers specific plans to help you either to moderate your drinking or to stop drinking entirely. Because many people first want to try to moderate their drinking, or need to try this before considering abstinence, these strategies will be presented first (chapters 7–9). If instead you decide that you would do better by learning how to abstain completely from alcohol, or if your attempt to moderate your drinking is not successful, turn to the techniques that will teach you how to stop drinking (chapters 10–13).

WHAT IF YOU NEED TREATMENT OR
WANT OUTSIDE HELP?

For a number of reasons, some people want outside help or discover that, despite their best efforts, they need the assistance of others. In the final four chapters, I offer advice for those seeking treatment, and I review the variety of treatment options that are available to you to help you make the best choice. Being an informed consumer and being able to ask the right questions will help you to get the help you need—if that is necessary.

A FINAL NOTE

This book is the result of many years of experience successfully working with people who have suffered from their alcohol consumption. This book is also based upon an extensive study of alcohol use, abuse, and treatment. It is true that some of what I say in this book is controversial. Not all professionals or paraprofessionals who work in the field agree with everything presented here. But my suggestions are not any less valid because of this, and they can help you if you heed them, work hard, and are honest with yourself. As you read this book, remember that your strong commitment to change is essential and that you must never lose sight of this.

Let your journey begin.

PART I

MAKING SENSE OF YOUR SITUATION

1

DO YOU HAVE
A DRINKING PROBLEM?

You can never learn less, you can only learn more.
R. BUCKMINSTER FULLER

Making the commitment to look at yourself and your relationship to alcohol is difficult. No one wants to admit that their drinking might be a problem. In some sectors of society, there is a stigma attached to having an alcohol problem, and you may feel that there is something wrong with you because you cannot always control your drinking. Drinking also probably plays an important role in your lifestyle, and most of your social activities may revolve around drinking. There is a part of you that loves to drink, whether it is the taste, the excitement, the feeling you get from alcohol, the social lubricant it provides, the relaxation, the pain it masks, or some other desire that fuels your drinking. The reason you are thinking about your drinking comes not from your sudden dislike for alcohol. It is because your drinking is causing you problems.

This is an important distinction that I will review in more detail in chapter 3. For now, keep in mind that your decision to look more closely at your drinking probably has little if anything to do with your wish to drink. You love to drink, and in the best of all worlds, you would continue to drink as you always have. If your drinking caused no problems, you would not even consider changing how you drink. Eliminating the problems that arise from your drinking is the reason you have arrived at this crossroads.

People who go on diets do not choose to eat less or different kinds of food because they no longer like to eat. They would love to continue to eat the way they always have! Rather, they choose to eat differently because they are sick and tired of being overweight. It is the consequences of eating too much that make them decide to eat differently.

Or take the person who has a gambling problem who makes the decision to stop gambling. This decision isn't made because the individual no longer likes gambling and the excitement it provides. People who gamble too much love to gamble! People make the decision to no longer gamble because gambling is causing significant destruction to their lives.

Obviously, you need to decide whether you even have a drinking problem. There is a fine line between a heavy social drinker and a problem drinker. Two common views about what describes a person with an alcohol-use problem are, first, the inability to predict what will happen when you drink and, second, continuing to drink despite the harmful consequences of your drinking. When reading these, think about your past drinking experiences and be totally honest with yourself. Consider whether any of the examples apply to you.

THE INABILITY TO PREDICT
WHAT WILL HAPPEN WHEN YOU DRINK

A person is believed to have a drinking problem if that person cannot *always* and *consistently* predict how much he or she will drink and what will happen once drinking begins. Individuals who fit this example drink regularly and generally without difficulty yet they sometimes or often

— stay out later than intended, and this causes an argument with a spouse, girlfriend, boyfriend, or another significant other;

— go to a bar with others to have just one or two drinks, but continue drinking for hours and become very drunk;

— become mean and obnoxious because of their drinking;

— miss work, school, or another important commitment due to hangovers;

— drink too much, which causes shame and embarrassment;

— regret something that was done or said while intoxicated;

— feel so physically bad the day after drinking that the day is wasted; or

— drink so much that they can't remember what happened or how they got home.

It is not that you always drink too much, but that you can't *consistently avoid* drinking too much. Often your drinking may be in control and may not cause you any difficulties, but at other times you drink too much, and there is a pattern of experiencing problems due to your drinking.

Tom is a 34-year-old married man and the father of 1-year-old twins. He had been a heavy social drinker while he was single. He had spent most weekends, and occasional weekdays, at bars with his high school friends. Since getting married at age 29, he purposely slowed down his drinking because his wife, Sally, wasn't into the bar scene. He was able to limit his drinking on most occasions, but occasionally when he went out without Sally, he found himself staying at the bar until very late at night and getting intoxicated, even though he had told Sally that he would be home after only a couple of drinks. He was able to limit his over-drinking episodes to only about once per month, but this pattern was beginning to affect his marriage. And despite his repeated attempts not to let this happen, it still did—over and over again. Tom just couldn't *consistently* and *reliably* control his drinking.

Another example is Kim, a 37-year-old woman who has been married to Jeff for eight years. Over the years, Kim and Jeff seemed to drift away from each other, at least in part because they didn't openly communicate with each other about some issues that were going on in their relationship. Kim generally would get home from work well before Jeff, who would often see some friends after work and not get home until much later. Whether due to Jeff's late arrivals or not, Kim got into a pattern of drinking wine when making dinner. While on most occasions Kim controlled her alcohol intake, several times each month Kim drank too much and was quite intoxicated when Jeff got home. Not only did this cause tension in the relationship, but when Kim was intoxicated, she would express her anger, which caused even more difficulties. And in spite of numerous promises and attempts not to over-drink, Kim still did, which resulted in even more tension and conflict.

It's Time to Be Honest with Yourself

Think about yourself and be completely honest. Do any of the examples listed on page 5 or do the cases of Tom or Kim describe your responses to alcohol? However hard you have tried to avoid problems as a result of drinking, have serious problems arisen anyway? If you answer yes, then you clearly need to address your drinking. This is true regardless of excuses such as "I hadn't eaten anything all day," or "I don't drink that much most of the time," or "I hadn't been out in months."

HARMFUL CONSEQUENCES RELATED TO DRINKING

People who continue to consume alcohol in spite of the harmful consequences related to drinking have a drinking problem. These consequences can affect their professional, social, legal, physical, or financial life. People who fall into this category continue to drink even though they

— spend so much money on alcohol that there is not enough money for other things;

— obtain information from a physician that their liver is in trouble because of consuming too much alcohol;

— argue or fight with a spouse, girlfriend, or boyfriend about their alcohol consumption;

— miss work or school due to their alcohol consumption;

— lose a job because of their drinking;

— alienate friends and family because of their drinking; or

— get arrested or involved with legal difficulties because of alcohol.

Chantal, a woman I counseled after she was arrested for drunk driving for the second time, is a 24-year-old single woman who first started drinking when she was 16. She states that she always loved the taste of alcohol and the feeling it gave her. She had fun with it and was never concerned about her drinking. She drank three or four times each week with her friends. She never experienced any problems related to alcohol until she was in her early 20s, when she was arrested for drunk driving. Still she didn't think alcohol was a problem and attributed her arrest to a case of bad luck and being in the wrong place at the wrong time.

Over the next several years, Chantal's drinking escalated, and she now admits that she lost several boyfriends due to her drinking. When drunk, she became flirtatious, and when confronted by her boyfriends got very angry and defensive, which eventually ended the relationships. Her drinking caused problems with some of her girlfriends as well. When intoxicated, Chantal's behavior and attitude changed, and she became argumentative and nasty. She eventually was again arrested for drunk driving, which finally led her to admit that she had a drinking problem.

Analyzing Your Relationship with Alcohol

Does Chantal's situation or do any of the statements listed on page 7 describe your experiences? The important point to remember in assessing a drinking problem is the *quality* of your drinking rather than the absolute *quantity* of alcohol you consume. The interaction between you and alcohol is what makes alcohol consumption a problem or not.

For example, if you drink only once or twice a year but it causes problems, then drinking is a problem. On the other hand, if you drink almost daily but your drinking has never caused you or anyone one else any concerns, then you may not have an alcohol problem.

The criteria for deciding whether you have a drinking problem are what happens when you drink and what problems alcohol causes you. If you can be totally honest with yourself, it is not difficult to decide whether drinking is a problem for you.

TAKING THE TEST

The MAST

Questionnaires have been developed to help people to assess whether alcohol use is a problem. One is the MAST, or the Michigan Alcoholism Screening Test, on pp. 10–11. Take this test *now, before* reading the next two paragraphs, and honestly answer the 25 questions.

To score this test, give yourself two points for each "no" answer to questions 1, 4, 6, and 8. For the rest of the questions, give yourself two points for each question you answered "yes," except give yourself only one point to questions 3, 5, 10, and 17, but five points for questions 9, 20, and 21. And don't score question 7 regardless of how you answer it; it was determined that this question wasn't helpful in determining who had an alcohol problem and who did not. Based upon the score, a person can be classified as not having a problem (0–3), maybe having a problem (3–4), or probably having a problem (5 and above).

How did you do? Based upon your score, do you think that you might need to do something about your drinking? If you earned at least five points, your drinking is a problem.

THE MICHIGAN ALCOHOLISM SCREENING TEST

1. Do you feel you are a normal drinker? Yes No
2. Have you ever awakened in the morning after some drinking the night before and found that you could not remember part of the evening? Yes No
3. Does your wife/husband or parents ever worry or complain about your drinking? Yes No
4. Can you stop drinking without a struggle after one or two drinks? Yes No
5. Do you ever feel bad about your drinking? Yes No
6. Do your friends or relatives think that you are a normal drinker? Yes No
7. Do you ever try to limit your drinking to certain times of the day or to certain places? Yes No
8. Are you always able to stop when you want to? Yes No
9. Have you ever attended a meeting of Alcoholics Anonymous? Yes No
10. Have you gotten into fights when drinking? Yes No
11. Has drinking ever created problems with you and your wife (husband)? Yes No
12. Has your wife (husband, or other family members) ever gone to anyone for help about your drinking? Yes No
13. Have you ever lost friends or girlfriends/boyfriends because of your drinking? Yes No
14. Have you ever gotten into trouble at work because of drinking? Yes No
15. Have you ever lost a job because of drinking? Yes No
16. Have you ever neglected your obligations, your family or work for two days or more in a row because of drinking? Yes No
17. Do you ever drink before noon? Yes No
18. Have you ever been told you have liver trouble? Yes No
19. Have you ever had DTs (delirium tremens), severe shaking, heard voices, or seen things that weren't there after heavy drinking? Yes No
20. Have you ever gone to anyone for help about your drinking? Yes No
21. Have you ever been in a hospital because of drinking? Yes No
22. Have you ever been a patient in a psychiatric hospital or a psychiatric ward of a general hospital where drinking was part of the problem? Yes No

continued on next page

23. Have you ever been at a psychiatric or mental health clinic, or gone to a doctor or clergyman for help with an emotional problem in which drinking has played a part?   Yes   No
24. Have you ever been arrested, even for a few hours, because of drunken behavior?   Yes   No
25. Have you ever been arrested for drunken driving or driving after drinking?   Yes   No

Reprinted with permission from the *American Journal of Psychiatry,* © 1971 American Psychiatric Association.

The CAGE

Another simple screening tool is called the CAGE, which you can take now.

THE CAGE

Have you ever felt that you should **C**ut down on your drinking?

Have people **A**nnoyed you by criticizing your drinking?

Have you ever felt bad or **G**uilty about your drinking?

Have you ever had a drink the first thing in the morning to "steady your nerves" or get rid of a hangover (**E**yeopener)?

So, how did you do on the CAGE? Did you answer "yes" to any of these questions? If you did, your drinking is causing you problems.

Even though questionnaires of this kind can be helpful, they are not as important as truthfully looking at yourself. You don't need a questionnaire to know if you are overweight, if you are happy with your job, or if you are satisfied with your financial situation. Likewise, you don't need a questionnaire to determine whether drinking is an issue for you. If you have the courage to be honest with yourself, you won't need a paper-and-pencil test to decide if you have a problem with alcohol.

BUT I'M NOT THAT BAD!

Maybe you found when you took these tests and honestly looked at yourself that your drinking does affect you and others, but that you still function pretty well. You discovered that while alcohol does cause you some problems, you aren't that bad. You still work every day, meet your financial obligations, and are generally successful. In fact, you know others who have a much more serious alcohol problem than you have. You need to know that

- Most people who struggle with the consequences of drinking continue to work and meet their financial obligations.
- They do not drink every day and, in many ways, they continue to hold up most of their responsibilities.
- They are often very successful in many realms of their lives.
- The image of the skid-row drunk represents only a very small percentage of people who have a serious alcohol problem.

Remember: Although alcohol may not affect every aspect of your life, it can still clearly cause damage to your life. Don't allow the thought "I am not that bad" prevent you from doing something about your drinking.

BE HONEST WITH YOURSELF

If your drinking causes you and others around you serious difficulties, you have an alcohol use problem. It is just that simple. If you have any doubts, reread this chapter. And remember that you do not need to experience all of these difficulties to conclude that you have a drinking problem. Even occasional problems that happen over and over again qualify. Only your honest evaluation of past drinking and its effect on your life can lead you forward. If you are truthful with yourself, you will have no difficulty deciding whether your alcohol consumption is something you need to address, either by learning to drink moderately or by complete abstinence from alcohol.

If you conclude that you have a problem with alcohol, you may wonder, "Why does drinking cause *me* problems, while others seem to be able to drink moderately and without any difficulty?" "Why am I different?" "Why do I drink too much?" "Why can't I drink like others do?" or "What is wrong with me?"

There are two basic perspectives to help you to answer these questions: the disease perspective and the learned behavior perspective. There is also one perspective that you should not consider: the personal weakness perspective. The next chapter will help you to understand yourself, and that understanding will determine how you will deal with your problem, now that you know you have one.

2

WHY DOES DRINKING
CAUSE YOU DIFFICULTY?

*There are no eternal facts as there are no absolute
truths.*   FRIEDRICH NIETZSCHE

Okay. So you have honestly looked at yourself and realize that your
drinking is hurting you. Maybe you don't always run into trouble
when you drink, but this often happens, and you have noticed a
destructive pattern. The next question is "Why?" Why can't you
consistently control your consumption of alcohol? What is wrong
with you? Why you can't drink like others who don't experience
problems when they drink?

Some people may wonder whether they are an *alcoholic,* whatever
that word really means. So often, after it becomes clear that a person I
see has a problem with alcohol, they either want to know if they are an
alcoholic or they say something like this to me: "I know I have a
problem with drinking, but I am not an *alcoholic,*" as if it is a dirty
word. I have seen heated discussions between spouses, when a wife, for
example, accuses her husband of being an alcoholic, and the husband

vehemently denies it. I have also met people who find that acknowl-edging that they are alcoholic provides them with relief and comfort.

In this chapter, to help you to understand and make sense of your situation, I will review the two main perspectives on why some peo-ple have a problem with alcohol. This understanding will help you to develop a course of action. Before I do this, though, I will first describe a point of view that is prevalent in society but that is not true and that you should not hold. This perspective is destructive, and if you already believe it, you should dispel it from your mind.

THE PERSONAL WEAKNESS PERSPECTIVE

Society often believes that there is something abnormal about people who drink too much. Unlike "normal" healthy people who drink without difficulty, people who over-drink do not control their alco-hol use, and they allow their use of alcohol to get the best of them. The inability to control alcohol intake is believed to stem from some kind of personal weakness. This idea may not be outwardly ver-balized, but the belief exists.

The main argument in this perspective focuses on "choice." It is believed that people "choose" whether to drink too much. And if they "choose" to drink too much and cause problems for themselves, others, and society, it is maintained that these people are irresponsible and lacking in some way. It follows that they must be weak people because they do not control their use of alcohol. The social stigma re-lated to having an alcohol abuse problem originates from this belief.

An Illogical Idea

Although the personal weakness perspective is popular in many seg-ments of our society, there is a huge logical problem with this point of view: *many, many people who have a drinking problem show incredible strength and fortitude in other areas of their lives.* For example, many successful business people, professional athletes, physicians, and entertainers have or have had a drinking problem. These people have demonstrated a powerful will to succeed and have shown personal determination in many aspects of their lives. It is hard to make sense of this if all individuals who have a drinking problem are weak people.

Also, lots of people who have messed up their lives as a result of alcohol one day resolve their drinking problem and see their lives begin to flourish and blossom. They achieve what they want to and become successful. If they were truly weak people, this simply wouldn't be possible.

Human Nature

It is human nature for people to struggle with the inability to control their behavior at some time in their lives. For example, common problems include being unable to control aggression, feeling anxious about speaking in front of an audience, being afraid to speak one's mind in a conflict situation, overworking, or compulsive exercising, to name just a few. If we do not consider these people weak or lacking in character strength, you should not consider yourself weak or lacking in character strength just because you have a drinking problem.

Nearly everyone can get stuck in a certain way of being in the world. Sigmund Freud, the father of psychoanalysis, noted this over a hundred years ago. He found that people often repeat the same behavior over and over again, despite suffering from adverse consequences. Freud named this the "repetition compulsion." Struggling with an alcohol problem is one way of being stuck, not necessarily a sign of being weak or defective in some way.

A Dangerous Trap

Don't buy into the personal weakness point of view. The worst thing you can do is "beat yourself up" for drinking too much or believe that you are a weak person because you drink too much. This will only make you feel worse about who you are and will damage your sense of self. In fact, you may even fall into the trap of drinking more to cope with feeling so bad. This is why the personal weakness perspective is so destructive.

Rather than viewing yourself as weak, it is important that you see yourself as having a drinking problem caused by a variety of complex factors that you do not fully understand. Consider that your drinking is your way of coping with forces just beyond your grasp. You are no different from people who struggle with other problems in their lives. Perhaps you need to develop new coping skills and ideas about yourself, which may include viewing your problem with alcohol a little differently.

THE DISEASE PERSPECTIVE

The most widely held understanding about an alcohol problem throughout Western culture is that it is a disease. The name given to this disease is *alcoholism*. The idea that a drinking problem is a disease is believed by the American Medical Association, American Psychiatric Association, American Public Health Association, American Hospital Association, American Psychological Association, National Association of Social Workers, World Health Organization, American College of Physicians, and American Society of Addiction Medicine.

So what does it mean that a drinking problem is a disease? According to *Webster's Dictionary,* a disease is a condition of the body or one of its parts that impairs the performance of a vital function. Clearly, while under the influence of alcohol, the brain is not functioning well. Also, over time, alcohol can damage most every organ in your body. Calling a drinking problem a disease does not, however, describe what the disease is all about or what causes it.

You're Born with It

For many, the disease of alcoholism is an inherited, biological vulnerability that predisposes a person to develop a problem with alcohol. This biological vulnerability interacts with a person's living situation, culture, and emotions and causes the person to drink too much. From this perspective, it is not the alcoholic's fault that he or she cannot drink responsibly and with control. Such individuals have an illness that makes them unable to handle their liquor and drink in moderation. Although the mechanism by which this happens is not completely understood, for them, even one drink may lead to a loss of control over their drinking. That is, one drink will lead to more drinking, and eventually, the use of alcohol becomes uncontrolled and takes over the person.

The Disease Is Chronic, Progressive, and Fatal

- Chronic: It is always there. You have it for life and it doesn't go away.
- Progressive: It will get worse and worse over time if left untreated.
- Fatal: You can die from it if it is left untreated.

F. Scott Fitzgerald wrote, "First you take a drink, then the drink takes a drink, then the drink takes you." In other words, drinking can take over your life, and eventually, it can kill you.

Alcoholism through the Ages

The idea that excessive drinking may be a disease was first noted over two hundred years ago.

- In the late 1700s to the early 1800s, Dr. Benjamin Rush, whom the Temperance Movement (1845–1918) claimed as its founder, was among the first to write about it. He wrote that while drinking was first the effect of "free agency," eventually the habit turned into a necessity and was a "disease of the will." He also prescribed abstinence as the only cure.

- In 1838, Samuel B. Woodward, superintendent of a mental asylum in Worcester, Massachusetts, and perhaps the leading mental health physician of the time, wrote a series of articles that described alcohol addiction as a "physical disease." He also wrote that the desire for alcohol could be so uncontrollable that it was questionable whether the power of the will could fight the desire to drink.

- In the early 1900s, the idea that alcoholism was a disease continued to be accepted within the psychiatric and social work field, although the specifics of it had not been fully worked out. It is fair to say, though, that the cause of alcoholism was believed to be alcohol, due to its power to take over the will of the person.

- In the 1930s and 1940s, ideas about the cause of alcoholism began to shift. With the renewed interest in alcohol problems in the United States, in large part due to the development of AA and the Yale Center of Alcohol Studies, researchers started to revise their understanding and began to believe that the disease of alcoholism was something that occurred only to some people for unclear reasons.

- In 1960, E. M. Jellinek, the founder of the Center of Alcohol Studies and Summer School of Alcohol Studies, originally at Yale and now at Rutgers University, published his book, *The Disease Concept of Alcoholism,* which outlined the medical model of alcoholism. He identified several different types of alcoholics. According to him, some of these individuals experienced a "loss of control," in which any drinking began a chain reaction that led to more and more drinking, which made it impossible to control alcohol intake. He also noted that the cause of some types of alcoholism may be inherited.

- In 1976, The American Society of Addiction Medicine (ASAM), the leading group of physicians in the United States dedicated to the understanding and treatment of substance abuse problems, developed a definition of alcoholism that stated it was a disease.

- In 1990, ASAM modified their definition of alcoholism to state that heredity was involved and that alcoholism was an involuntary disability marked by the inability to consistently control drinking.

Is a Drinking Problem an Inherited Condition?

Is it possible that your heredity could be responsible for your over-drinking? And if this is true, how does your genetic makeup play a role? These are complicated questions, and there is still much that we have to learn. But let me tell you what is currently known.

First, it is clear that heredity is important. We know that children of alcoholic parents who are adopted at birth and raised in non-alcoholic families have a much greater rate of developing alcoholism than children of nonalcoholic parents who are adopted at birth and raised by alcoholic parents. So heredity is important, even more than the environment in which one grows up.

One study followed a group of adolescent boys for about 40 years. The adolescents were given a variety of psychological tests, and their families were also assessed. As these individuals matured, some developed serious problems with alcohol, and others did not. It was found that the rate of serious alcohol problems among men who had two or more alcohol-abusing relatives was about three times higher than among men who had no alcohol-abusing relatives. In fact, one of the best predictors of developing a problem with alcohol is coming from a family in which one or more members have had a problem with alcohol. In most cases, people I have seen who struggle with alcohol report that biological relatives have drinking problems.

Studies of twins have also shown that genes are important by comparing the rates of alcohol problems among identical twins with the rates of alcohol problems among fraternal twins. Identical twins share the same genes, but fraternal twins do not. Therefore, if alcohol problems are largely biologically determined, both members of a set of identical twins will more often have alcohol problems, than will both members of a set of fraternal twins.

Again, the results were very clear: there is a higher rate of alcohol problems among identical twins than among fraternal twins, which supports the idea that alcohol problems are at least in part biologically and genetically determined.

How Does Heredity Increase the Risk of
Developing an Alcohol Problem?

So if heredity is responsible for developing a problem with alcohol, how does this work? What is it about what is inherited that causes a person to over-drink?

Very often, children of parents who have alcohol problems, who presumably have a biological vulnerability to develop a problem themselves, feel less intoxicated when they drink the same amount of alcohol as people with no family history of drinking problems. Alcohol simply affects them less, and they can drink a lot without feeling particularly intoxicated. It follows that this ability to handle alcohol, which is biologically based and inherited, may lead them to drink more than others to obtain the same effect from alcohol. This leads to increased rates of drinking and drinking problems.

The "Hollow Leg" Syndrome

You may have heard of the "hollow leg" syndrome, in which some people seem to be able to put away huge quantities of alcohol in their "hollow leg" without showing signs of gross intoxication. I am sure that you know what this is like. You are probably able to drink a lot more than some other people you know who get drunk after only a few drinks. While some people consider this a source of pride and sign of personal strength, in truth, it is really a sign of a potential drinking problem.

People with different responses to alcohol have been studied over many years to see if those who can drink a lot without feeling intoxicated have a greater chance of developing alcohol problems. Once again, the evidence is clear: people who have a low response to alcohol have a much greater chance of becoming alcoholic compared to people who get intoxicated after only one or two drinks.

Nothing Happens in a Vacuum

We should also remember that the genetic susceptibility passed from parent to child must interact with psychological, social, and cultural factors in order to result in an alcohol problem. For example, you might have a biological vulnerability to develop a drinking problem, but if you live in a society where drinking is frowned upon and discouraged or where alcohol simply is not available, you probably will never develop a drinking problem because you choose not to or cannot drink. On the other hand, if you are biologically vulnerable and you live in an environment where heavy drinking is common, developing a problem with alcohol is very likely. So, the development of an alcohol problem is very complicated. Regardless, the drinking-as-a-disease perspective places a heavy emphasis on heredity to understand why people cannot consistently control their drinking.

So What Does This Mean for You?

It Isn't Your Fault. The drinking-as-a-disease perspective doesn't blame you or anyone for having an alcohol problem. It is not your fault that drinking cannot be controlled, because how your body reacts to alcohol is largely genetically determined. This perspective also emphasizes the importance of compassion for the problem drinker rather than degradation. If we know anything, it is that support and compassion help people who drink too much.

Drinking Can't Be Controlled. If someone has the disease of alcoholism, drinking can't be controlled. This loss of control is inevitable and largely defines the nature of the beast. No matter how hard you try, you will always drink too much. So, the only way to resolve the problem is by not drinking at all and never taking that first drink.

There Is No Going Back. If a person has the disease of alcoholism, there is no going back. There is an expression that once a cucumber changes into a pickle, the pickle can never go back to being a cucumber. Well, the same is true about alcoholism. Once a person becomes alcoholic, that person can't ever go back to being a social drinker. Once this line is crossed, people must accept their condition and learn that they cannot drink safely.

No matter how hard you have tried to control your drinking, has your drinking escalated and have you eventually returned to your old habits and problems? Do you think that you have the disease of alcoholism? If you do, abstinence is the only way to overcome your illness. There is no alternative, and this is your only solution.

THE LEARNED BEHAVIOR PERSPECTIVE

Human beings are creatures of learning. We learn how to walk, how to read, how to write, how to golf, how to swim, and how to play tennis. We also learn how to avoid pain, how to obtain pleasure, what makes us happy, and what makes us sad. We learn what kinds of food we like and what kinds of food we dislike. We learn the type of people we like to be with and, as important, the type of people we don't want to be around. And we even learn how to drink alcohol.

When I talk with people who struggle with drinking, I am always very interested in how they discovered alcohol, what they like about drinking, and what influences played a role in how they learned to drink. Did they grow up in a household where alcohol flowed freely? Were many, if not most, of their peers into the heavy drinking scene? Was drinking to get drunk the norm in their immediate surroundings? Was it common to unwind after work by drinking? In some cultures, drunkenness is tolerated, if not encouraged, but in other societies, heavy drinking is discouraged. All of these influences play a role in how people learn to use alcohol.

Over the course of their lives, people learn how alcohol makes them feel, and some learn to use alcohol to enhance or take away certain feelings. For example, some people use alcohol as a way to decrease tension and stress. Others use it as a social lubricant that helps them to feel more relaxed around others. Some may have discovered that alcohol helps them to feel less depressed or gives them energy. And some people learned that alcohol takes away their boredom and loneliness.

The learned behavior perspective maintains that, to a large degree, excessive drinking is unhealthy learned behavior. While this perspective may accept that some people have a greater chance of developing a problem with alcohol than others due to their heredity, this perspective still views a drinking problem as largely being learned.

Learned Behavior or a Disease—Who Cares?

So what does it matter if a drinking problem is learned behavior as opposed to a disease? It is important because the perspective that a drinking problem is learned behavior allows for the possibility that a person with a drinking problem may be able to learn to drink differently . . . and to drink less. If problem drinking is learned, it may be possible for some people to learn how to moderate their drinking. This is in contrast to the drinking-as-a-disease perspective, which maintains that it is simply not possible for an alcoholic to drink differently. The only way to resolve a drinking problem from the disease perspective is via complete and total abstinence from alcohol.

So Can a Pickle Be Turned Back into a Cucumber?

Although the drinking-as-a-disease perspective says it isn't possible, some people who have experienced a drinking problem have been able to change their pattern of alcohol use and have learned to drink differently. When people change their pattern of drinking, this change can take any number of forms, including

— drinking extremely occasionally, such as only on holidays or at special events;

— totally abstaining from alcohol for a period of time, but eventually starting to do some limited drinking again;

— limiting drinking to only weekends and drinking only a few drinks;

— drinking only in social settings when they know they won't overdo it;

— drinking several times per week, but limiting the amount they drink; or

— changing the type of alcohol they drink.

Less important than how they are doing it is the simple fact that they are *able* to do this, which suggests that maybe a drinking problem is largely learned and that people can learn to drink differently and without problems.

The Rand Report

Perhaps one of most famous studies that showed that some problem drinkers could learn to drink differently was a study known as the Rand Report. The study examined over 900 males who struggled with drinking and who had been treated in 45 alcohol treatment programs across the United States. These treatment programs all maintained that abstinence was the only way to resolve a drinking problem. In spite of this treatment orientation, one-and-a-half years later it was found that a significant number of these people were drinking moderately, at amounts that couldn't be understood as destructive or as out of control.

While one and one-half years is not that long, this was a very large, well-designed study that challenged conventional wisdom that people who struggled with drinking would *immediately* resume out-of-control drinking after taking that first drink. However, other, smaller studies have followed people with significant alcohol problems for many years and have found the same thing—that some people with drinking problems are able to learn how to control their drinking. Perhaps some pickles can be turned back into cucumbers.

Can Old Dogs Be Taught New Tricks?

The Rand Report and other studies showed that old dogs can, by themselves, learn new tricks. Although the treatment offered focused on abstinence, many people instead learned to control their drinking. But can people who struggle with alcohol be taught to drink less? The drinking-as-learned-behavior perspective holds that if drinking is learned, treatment that focuses on teaching people how to drink less should be successful. And in fact, many people who have suffered from drinking too much have been taught to drink less with treatment that uses principles of learning.

What Does This Mean for You?

The drinking-as-learned-behavior perspective suggests that not all people who have an alcohol problem have the disease alcoholism and must abstain from alcohol to stop alcohol from ruining their lives. This perspective questions the whole concept that a drinking problem is a disease. While heredity is relevant, this perspective tends to view an alcohol problem as maladaptive learned behavior that results from a variety of sources: psychological, social, cultural, and educational. While abstinence may be the best policy for many, this perspective suggests that there is a place for the individual who may be able to successfully learn how to moderate drinking.

SO WHAT IS THE TRUTH?

So what is the truth? Should you view your problem as a disease or as an unhealthy learned habit? This is a complicated question that only you can answer.

There Are Many Truths

I believe that the cause of an alcohol problem is very complex and that there are different truths for different people. An alcohol problem can be caused by biological, psychological, or cultural factors, to name just a few, or by a combination of all of these. It is shortsighted and narrow-minded to think that there is only one way to understand a person's problem with alcohol.

Find Your Own Truth

How you understand your problem with alcohol is a decision that only you can make, and your belief must benefit you and no one else. If you believe that your drinking problem is the result of a disease, then view it this way. For many individuals, the idea that they have a disease works because it provides a clear road to recovery. Because having a disease implies that you are not at fault, you may overcome any guilt (which you should not have anyway) as well.

I have seen many people who had very destructive patterns of drinking, began drinking problematically at an early age, and reported that drinking problems ran heavily in their families. They had repeatedly tried to moderate their drinking without success and could offer no explanation for why they could not control their drinking other than "I am an alcoholic." The idea of having a disease was the only way they could understand themselves, and it fit for them.

I am reminded of Mitchell, who told me that from the time he first tasted alcohol he was a "blackout" drinker. He would drink to get drunk, and he would often experience blackouts in which he couldn't remember what he had done the night before or how he got home. As an adult, if he drank, he would binge drink until he was so physically ill that he couldn't drink anymore. The only way Mitchell could understand himself was that he had the disease of alcoholism. He knew that if he continued to drink, he would eventually die from it.

On the other hand, you may want to view your drinking as a bad habit or as something you have learned, whether the reasons are psychological, cultural, or social. The idea of being diseased or alcoholic may not sit well with you. Having a disease may make you feel defective or abnormal. You may think that you could learn to control your drinking, and you may want to try.

However, even if you don't accept the idea that you have a disease, you can still choose abstinence to solve your problem. Certainly, I have worked with people who could never "buy" the disease perspective, yet who still chose to totally abstain from alcohol as the way to recover from their drinking problem. I am reminded of Sam, age 45, a successful individual who drank heavily and almost daily in his youth. Over time, he was able to limit his drinking to only a few times a year. However, every time he drank, he experienced difficulties. He finally chose abstinence as the way to recover from his problem, but he always understood his problem as a bad habit rather than as a disease.

How you perceive your drinking problem must fit with your view of the world. How you choose to view your alcohol problem must help you and no one else. There aren't any right or wrong answers, unless your answers lead to more drinking problems.

The most significant issue is not what you call your drinking problem or how you see it, but making the decision to do something about your drinking and implementing a plan of action.

PART II
BEFORE YOU GET STARTED

3

GETTING READY AND STAYING MOTIVATED

A person with half volition goes backwards and forwards, but makes no progress on even the smoothest of roads.   THOMAS CARLYLE

It's not that some people have willpower and some don't. It's that some people are ready to change and others are not.   JAMES GORDON, M.D.

Things do not change. We change.

HENRY DAVID THOREAU

By now you have enough information to know that you have a problem with alcohol. You have honestly evaluated your situation and you have reached the conclusion that your use of alcohol is causing you difficulty in one or more areas of your life. You may also have given a name to your problem with alcohol, whether you call it a disease, an illness, or a bad habit. And you have learned that you should not beat yourself up for having an alcohol problem. You are no different than the person who struggles in other ways, such as an individual who can't always control his or her temper, stress level, or tendency to work too much. Things are somewhat out of control, and you are stuck in a pattern of behavior that is causing you distress.

However, that happens to most people in some way during the course of their lives.

As I stated in the first chapter, while it is difficult to look at your drinking and arrive at the realization that your use of alcohol is a problem, it is often even more difficult to make the decision to change your pattern of alcohol use and put a plan into action. You enjoy many things about drinking despite the fact that drinking also hurts you. You may enjoy how drinking makes you feel, the social aspects of drinking, the way it relaxes you, the taste, or the fun it provides you. At the same time, you may occasionally not like how you act when you drink too much, or how drinking negatively affects your relationship with your wife, husband, girlfriend, or boyfriend, how it hurts you financially, or how drinking too much makes you feel the next day. However, not wanting to give up the positive aspects of drinking can make it hard to take action, can make you question your decision to change, and can play a role in leading you back to your old behaviors.

AMBIVALENCE

Ambivalence is having simultaneous and contradictory feelings or attitudes toward something, whether this is a person, object, or action. And this can lead to uncertainty about what course of action to take. As a result, movement doesn't occur, and you stay the present course. Ambivalence can keep a person stuck.

You should know that this is very different than not acknowledging that you have a problem. You may fully realize that drinking is a problem for you, yet you may not have made the decision to take action and change your relationship to alcohol. I have worked with many people who knew that their use of alcohol was a problem but were not ready to do the work to change their behavior. I have often heard things like this:

- "I am drinking too much, but I am not sure if I am ready to stop."
- "I don't know what to do. I know my drinking is hurting me, but I like it, too."
- "Boy, I know my drinking is damaging my relationship with my wife, but I enjoy drinking with my friends, and I don't know what I would do if I couldn't party with them."
- "Drinking is my downfall, but it is also my best friend."
- "I wish I would want to change. I know drinking is bad for me, but I just can't get up the desire to do something different and really change. I wish there was some kind of magic pill that I could take!"

Ambivalence can also lead you to slip back into your old ways. Mixed feelings can lead you to question yourself: "Why am I doing this?" "Do I really want to be doing this?" or "Do I really want to change?" I have certainly seen people who have made the decision to address their drinking problem but for whom, at some point, something changes. Their commitment begins to waver and they start to question themselves and their decision. For example, after deciding to no longer drink and successfully not drinking for several weeks, they may lose their commitment and start drinking again.

Ambivalence Is Universal

It is very common for people to know that they have a problem but not be ready to change, or after having made a decision to change, to lose their commitment and resume their old behaviors. For example, many people are overweight and realize that they need to lose weight but aren't ready to take the steps to begin a diet. They may not like the way they feel, their doctors may have strongly suggested that they lose weight, and they may not like the way they look. However, they love to eat and obtain many positive benefits from eating. They don't want to give up their favorite foods, or eat less, or give up the social aspects of eating. Despite the negative consequences of eating too much and being overweight, they fail to commit to action and change their eating habits. Or they begin a diet that starts well, but at some point they go off it and resume their out-of-control eating.

And what about cigarette smokers who fully know the dangers of smoking, can list many reasons for wanting to quit, and yet don't commit to stop smoking? Why don't they just stop? Apart from the physical withdrawal that can occur when someone stops smoking, there may be many other reasons for continuing to smoke, whether it is the relaxation smoking provides, the enjoyment of smoking, or even the fear of withdrawal, to name just a few factors that can prevent taking action. There are also smokers who joke, "It is easy to quit smoking. I have done it hundreds of times!" These people made the decision to stop smoking, but at some point their motivation faded away and they returned to smoking.

There are also people who are in a difficult relationship and just can't decide if they should leave their partner. While they may be very unhappy and can list numerous things they don't like about the person they're with, they also see positive aspects of staying the present course. They may like some things about their partner, or perhaps there are financial reasons for staying together. Their ambivalent feelings prevent them from taking action and keep them stuck. Some end up in a "ping-pong" type of relationship, breaking up and getting back together every few months due to their mixed feelings.

For some people, ambivalence results from a fear of changing and doing something different. While a part of them wants to change, and they can see benefits to changing, another part of them is too scared to take an unfamiliar path—like living life without alcohol. So they stay stuck and never quite put a plan of action into place.

Coming to Terms with Ambivalence

To develop and sustain a plan of action and change your behavior:

- Ambivalence must be overcome.
- An action plan must be put into place.
- You must stay on course.

Resolving ambivalence is absolutely essential if you are going to change your pattern of drinking. And the first step is to *become certain and remain certain* that the consequences of your drinking outweigh the advantages, or that the benefits of changing have a greater appeal than the drawbacks of changing. Whatever thrusts you into and keeps you on a course of action, the need to change must become and remain more important than staying the same.

Complete the Exercises

The *Pros and Cons of My Drinking* exercise on page 47 can help you come to terms with your ambivalence. Think carefully about what you like and don't like about your drinking. How does drinking help you, and how does drinking hurt you? Focus on your social life, your health, your financial situation, your work, your important relationships, any legal problems drinking may have caused you, and your self-esteem and emotional well-being. How does drinking impact any of these things, both in positive and negative ways?

Next, complete the *Pros and Cons of Changing* exercise on page 47. Think about the advantages changing your relationship to alcohol will offer and also think about the disadvantages of changing your drinking pattern. While there may be some overlap with the previous exercise, there can be some important differences, as the case of Mike shows.

Mike's drinking had for years had a negative impact on his relationship with Nancy, his wife. Over the years, Mike and Nancy had had numerous arguments about his drinking, but no screaming or pleading by Nancy about Mike's drinking ever made a difference. Mike primarily came to see me to placate Nancy. He knew his drinking was problematic, but he wasn't sure if he was truly ready to change it. He knew his drinking was destroying his marriage but seemed to accept this and really couldn't come up with any other harm that resulted from his drinking.

I asked Mike to complete the *Pros and Cons of My Drinking* exercise. He wrote down a number of pros, including

- "socializing with my friends"
- "relaxing"
- "love partying"

On the cons, the only thing he could come up with was

- "hurts my marriage"

Mike next completed the *Pros and Cons of Changing* exercise, and the first thing he wrote under the pros was

- "could get along with my wife and have fun again"

At that moment, I noticed a change in his demeanor and attitude, and I asked him about it. Mike stated that, while he always knew his drinking caused arguments between him and Nancy, he hadn't ever really thought much about how he could have a loving relationship with Nancy if he stopped drinking. That point, which should have been self-evident, somehow got lost in all of the arguing. Mike was flabbergasted by this realization, and it was the deciding factor that motivated him to change his pattern of drinking. For Mike, a perceived benefit of changing was a greater motivator than was a negative consequence of his drinking.

After completing these exercises, read each item you wrote and think about how important the particular consequences and benefits are for you. Focus on each reason until you have a clear sense of how important it is, and on a scale of 1–10, with 1 being very unimportant and 10 being very important, rank each item to see what reasons are most important for you. Often it is not the total number of reasons within a particular category that can help you to determine if you are ready to change, but one or more reasons that will really stick out as essential for you. In the previous example, Mike didn't even need to rank each of his reasons—he came to see what was most important to him spontaneously. This was not true for John.

John is a 38-year-old married man, the father of 7- and 10-year-old boys. In retrospect, he had had a drinking problem since his early 20s. He drank on most days, which caused daily arguments with his wife. He reported that this was affecting their relationship, and their yelling matches caused a lot of tension in the home. On the weekends, John drank more heavily, so much so that often an entire Sunday was blown as he slept off his hangover. John came to see me after he was arrested for drunk driving.

John admitted that he drank a fair amount and that drinking might be a problem for him, but he generally minimized the degree to which it caused him problems and affected his family. He understood his recent arrest as a case of being in the wrong place at the wrong time, but he also acknowledged that he often drove drunk and that this wasn't the best idea. He wasn't sure whether he was ready to change his relationship with alcohol.

I observed that John seemed to have some mixed feelings, and I asked him if he would complete the *Pros and Cons of My Drinking* and *Pros and Cons of Changing* exercises. On the *Pros and Cons of My Drinking* exercise, he wrote down many pros, including

- "seeing my friends"
- "It's fun."
- "I like the feeling."
- "I like the taste of beer."
- "It helps me to unwind."
- "I like the social scene."

The only cons he could come up with were:

- "getting arrested"
- "wife problems"

On the *Pros and Cons of Changing* exercise, the only pros John wrote were

- "won't ever get arrested again"
- "My wife would give me less grief."

He came up with many cons of changing, including

- "boredom"
- "not being able to see my friends"
- "missing the bar scene"
- "wouldn't be able to have fun"
- "couldn't unwind"

Before going through his list to see what was most important to John, I wanted to be sure that he covered all of the possible pros and cons. It seemed to me that some important things might be missing from his list—for example, there was nothing about his health or his children. I asked him about this, and with some exploration, he was able to acknowledge that his drinking was affecting his relationship with his children. He then wrote down under the cons of his drinking:

- "kids being afraid of me when I fight with my wife"
- "missing their hockey games on Sundays"

When I asked him if there would be any benefits to changing, he wrote

- "could have fun with my boys and see their hockey games"
- "kids wouldn't be afraid of me"

I then had John rank each item on his lists in order of importance. What John found was that all of the reasons that concerned his children were most important to him. While there were more reasons listed under the pros of drinking and the cons of changing, how his drinking hurt his relationship with his sons and how changing could improve their relationship led John to decide to change his pattern of drinking.

After you complete the exercise, review it *daily*. This will help you to keep focused on the problems your drinking has caused you and the positive things you will gain by changing your relationship to alcohol. It will reinforce your initial commitment to change and keep your motivation going.

Mixed Feelings Don't Just Evaporate

Most decisions we make in life aren't black or white. Even when we make a decision, some lingering mixed feelings are to be expected. For example, think about when we end a relationship or make a job change. While there are times when this decision is easy and clear, there are other times when we need to weigh the advantages and disadvantages of making a switch, and the decision is harder. However, at some point, the scales tip, and although we may have some mixed feelings, we reach and are able to make a decision.

The reasons and feelings that could keep you from putting an action plan into place or that could creep back into your mind to weaken your decision—the pros of drinking and the cons of changing —don't simply go away. *They can persist, but despite this, you can move forward anyway.*

Focus on the negative aspects of your drinking and the positive things you can get by changing, as opposed to the benefits of your drinking or the negative things about changing. The goal is that you will be able to realize that the reasons for changing outweigh and are more important to you than continuing to drink the way you have been.

Are You Still Not Sure?

After completing these exercises, you may find that the advantages of changing and the harmful consequences of your drinking don't outweigh the advantages of drinking and the disadvantages of changing.

Or you may see the need for change but may be scared to address your drinking, so much so that your fear prevents you from taking action. While you know that drinking is hurting you, there are things about drinking that you can't imagine not having, and these stop you from taking action. Maybe for you, ambivalence hasn't yet been resolved. You may still be thinking about changing and aren't yet ready to take control of your life and your drinking problem.

If you aren't sure whether the cons of drinking and the pros of changing outweigh the pros of drinking and the cons of changing:

- Make the commitment to change for a limited period of time to see what it is like. If you don't like it, you can always go back to the way you were. Thus, you have little to lose but much to gain. You owe it to yourself to at least experience something different, which may help you to make a longer-term decision. I am sure that you will find your life gets better once your drinking problem has been resolved.

If you are afraid to change your pattern of drinking:

- Remember that thinking about changing is scarier than actually doing it. In fact, this book will help you manage any fear you have, if that is a stumbling block. Don't let fear stand in your way. You will find that, when the time comes, you will be able to manage the things that once concerned you the most.

TWO OTHER MOTIVATION KILLERS

A Lack of Confidence or Learned Helplessness

It is possible that you don't begin a change process and take action because you don't have the confidence in yourself to change. As much as you want to be different, you don't believe in yourself and your abilities to make a change . . . so you simply don't try. You got the idea that you can't change because you previously tried to change and failed. As a result, you have resigned yourself to the fact that change is not possible. Believing, without proof and evidence, that you can't succeed has been called *learned helplessness.*

Learned helplessness has been documented in research using animals. In the original experiment, dogs were placed in a box and shocked, and the only way they could escape the shock was to jump over a barrier. After repeated shocks, the dogs learned to jump over the barrier. However, dogs that were placed in a box and couldn't escape getting shocked couldn't even be trained to avoid shock when escape was later made possible. Instead, they gave up and accepted the shock because they had previously learned there was nothing they could do to avoid it. They had *learned* that they were helpless.

This often happens with people who struggle with alcohol consumption. After many unsuccessful attempts at trying to quit drinking, they eventually give up, accept failure, and stop trying. They, too, have *learned* to be helpless.

Fortunately, the story of the helpless dogs doesn't end here. In another experiment, dogs that had accepted their fate and wouldn't escape the shock were finally trained to escape by being coaxed and forced by the researchers. After they were repeatedly pulled with a leash over the barrier while being shocked, the dogs eventually learned on their own to avoid the shock. With some outside prodding, they understood that they had control over their situation and were no longer helpless.

If a lack of confidence is stopping you:

• If you no longer believe that you can succeed, and *learned helplessness* plays a role in your inability to stop drinking, remember that past failure doesn't mean future failure. Don't allow the belief that you can't achieve success to become a self-fulfilling prophecy. Maybe you didn't go about it in the right way last time; learn from this rather than seeing yourself as someone who cannot change. Rarely has a person been completely successful at their first attempt to change, and this is particularly true for people who are trying to change their pattern of drinking. The dogs learned that they could change, and you, too, need to remember that change is always possible. The key is to never give up.

A Fear of Failing

Perhaps you do not want to risk failing, so you never put an action plan in place. Or if you've failed in the past, you are all too familiar with the disappointment of not succeeding and don't want to experience that again. So instead of trying and possibly having to face failure, you stay the present course.

If a fear of failing is stopping you:

• Stop viewing your past attempts to get a handle on your drinking as failures. Instead, see them as unsuccessful attempts and recognize that you simply haven't succeeded yet. Failure is an endpoint and only happens when you stop trying. So, if you continue to try, it can never be said that you failed. You just haven't succeeded . . . *yet.*

MOVING FORWARD

I hope, though, that you are not in any of these positions. You are reading this book, which means that you are concerned about your drinking and are seriously thinking of doing something about it. In truth, despite any feelings that can take you away from addressing your drinking, you obviously have some motivation to change because you are reading this book. This means that you are concerned about your drinking and are seriously thinking of doing something about it. Try to keep your mind focused on the consequences of your drinking and the benefits of changing, which will help you to stay on track.

> *There are risks and costs to a program of action,*
> *but they are far less than the long-range risks and*
> *costs of comfortable inaction.*   JOHN F. KENNEDY

> *Do the thing you fear to do and keep on doing it*
> *. . . that is the quickest and surest way ever yet*
> *discovered to conquer fear.*   DALE CARNEGIE

> *If you have no confidence in self, you are twice de-*
> *feated in the race of life. With confidence, you*
> *have won even before you have started.*
> MARCUS GARVEY

> *I am not judged by the number of times I fail, but*
> *by the number of times I succeed; and the number*
> *of times I succeed is in direct proportion to the*
> *number of times I can fail and keep on trying.*
> TOM HOPKINS

PROS AND CONS OF MY DRINKING

PROS OF MY DRINKING

Write down all of the things you like about drinking—think of your relationships, your emotional state, your social life, or anything else you like about drinking. When done, rank each item from 1–10, **with 1 being the least important and 10 being the most important.**

CONS OF MY DRINKING

Write down all of ways your drinking hurts you—think of your relationships, your health, your emotional state, your job or school, your finances, or any legal troubles. When done, rank each item from 1–10, **with 1 being the least important and 10 being the most important.**

PROS AND CONS OF CHANGING

PROS OF CHANGING

Write down all of the ways that changing your drinking pattern may help you—think of your relationships, your health, your emotional state, your job or school, your finances, or any legal troubles. When done, rank each item from 1–10, **with 1 being the least important and 10 being the most important.**

CONS OF CHANGING

Write down all of the ways that changing your drinking pattern may hurt you—think of your relationships, your emotional state, your social life, or any other thing that concerns you about changing your pattern of drinking. When done, rank each item from 1–10, **with 1 being the least important and 10 being the most important.**

4

CAN YOU REALLY
HELP YOURSELF?

Only I can change my life. No one can do it for me.
CAROL BURNETT

It is the truth we ourselves speak rather than the treatment we receive that heals us. HOBART MOWRER

By now, you have honestly evaluated your situation and you have decided that you must change your relationship to alcohol in order to lead a more satisfying life, one free from alcohol-related problems. The scales have tipped in favor of changing, and you are ready to develop a plan of action.

Yet quitting or cutting down is often difficult. Perhaps you have tried before—perhaps many times, or with treatment—only to return to your old ways. Having been unable to succeed, you may feel hopeless, dejected, frustrated, and angry.

On the other hand, perhaps this is the first time that you have been serious about doing something about your drinking. Regardless of your particular situation, you may be wondering what you can do to help yourself and whether you need to seek help such as AA meetings or substance abuse counseling.

SOME PEOPLE THINK THAT TREATMENT IS ESSENTIAL

Our society perpetuates the idea that no one's alcohol problem will go away without the support of a counselor, a treatment program, or a support group like AA. Advertisements for addiction treatment programs often assert that professional help is required. Statements such as "alcoholism is a treatable illness" or "alcohol problems do not go away if left untreated" dominate the social scene. In 1993, the former director of the National Institute of Drug Abuse, Robert Dupont, wrote: "Addiction is not self-curing. Left alone addiction only gets worse, leading to total degradation, to prison, and, ultimately to death." Also, as was discussed in chapter 2, the idea that a drinking problem is a disease is embraced by many people. If this is true, it follows that this disease requires treatment like other diseases.

These advertisements or the idea that a drinking problem is a disease may have caused you to think that no one with a drinking problem can possibly change his or her life without receiving treatment. We all know people—family, friends, and neighbors—who have tried unsuccessfully to stop drinking on their own, which could discourage you. Or you may believe or hear from others that unless a person gets involved in treatment, they are not really serious about helping themselves.

THE TRUTH ABOUT TREATMENT

Many, many individuals with a long history of alcohol abuse have resolved their drinking problems without attending AA or any other type of self-help meetings or ever receiving treatment from a therapist, counselor, or treatment program of any kind. Despite societal beliefs that people with alcohol problems must obtain treatment, it is clear that even individuals who struggle with severe alcohol problems can achieve recovery without treatment. The respected American Psychiatric Association and the Institute of Medicine state this as well.

WHAT RESEARCH SHOWS

During the past 50 years, there have been many reports of people who helped themselves with their drinking problems without treatment, either by abstaining from alcohol completely or by moderating their drinking. The first reports were generally cases of specific individuals who were able to do so. However, as research in this area has grown, studies have looked at larger populations of people. Some researchers studied people over time to see how alcohol problems progress with and without treatment; other researchers surveyed people to discover if they had a drinking problem, if they had resolved it, and if so, how.

Observing People over Time

Did people who received treatment for their drinking problems fare better over time than people who did not? What is interesting is that a study has found that there was essentially no difference in outcomes between the groups. Regardless of whether or not people received treatment, the same percentage got better each year. People seemed to heal themselves, as opposed to treatment being the deciding factor.

Surveys

Surveys that ask people if they ever suffered from an alcohol problem and if and how they resolved it have also found that many people with alcohol problems are able to help themselves. One study involved over 11,000 people who were asked about their drinking to determine their past and present use of alcohol. Of the people who said that they had resolved their problem for at least one year, 75 percent reported doing it without any kind of outside help or treatment.

Another study, sponsored by the National Institute on Alcohol Abuse and Alcoholism and called the National and Longitudinal Alcohol Epidemiologic Study (NLAES), conducted interviews with almost 43,000 adults over age 18 who lived throughout the United States. A lot of information was obtained, including about their alcohol use and related problems and any treatment they had received. Of the people interviewed, about 4,600 people had experienced a serious alcohol problem anywhere from 1 to 20 years before the interview.

Of those 4,600 people, about 25 percent had received treatment, and about 75 percent never received any type of treatment. Of the people who never received treatment of any kind, 74 percent were able to recover from their drinking problem.

DON'T SOME PEOPLE NEED TREATMENT?

Yes—there are two situations in which treatment is essential. Some people must be medically detoxified from their alcohol abuse. As you will read in the next chapter, it can be extremely dangerous for someone who is physiologically dependent upon alcohol to suddenly stop drinking without professional assistance. Some people who have a drinking problem have other serious difficulties in their lives, which can interfere with their ability to go it alone. These problems may include depression, unemployment and related stress, domestic violence, marital breakups, legal challenges, and others. Alcohol-abusing people with serious social or emotional difficulties will have more trouble getting a handle on their alcohol use without treatment and some kind of outside support. Such individuals should seek the help and guidance of trained substance abuse professionals.

However, even for people who need or want outside treatment, what they bring to treatment and their internal motivation and desire to change are critical for their success. Without commitment and hard work, treatment won't do much.

YOU CAN AND MUST HELP YOURSELF

The idea that the majority of people who struggle with alcohol consumption are able to help themselves without treatment fits with my experience. I have found that treatment is often the least important factor when a person resolves a drinking problem.

Over the years, I have spoken with numerous individuals with serious alcohol problems who had been admitted many times for detoxification to inpatient alcoholism treatment programs. Typically, shortly after being discharged they began to drink again, and within a fairly short period of time, they needed to be admitted once again. However, after being discharged one particular time, they remained abstinent. They were not sure what was different, but something "clicked." They finally were ready to get serious about ending their problem with alcohol. Whatever triggered the change, they had had enough.

As we talked, I was struck with how, at that moment of their decision, their mental state, not the treatment, had been the most important factor. It is even possible that, at that time, they would have achieved success without treatment, because they were simply ready to change their lives.

Suzie is a 59-year-old woman who has been abstinent from alcohol for the past 13 years. Suzie began drinking in her teenage years, and rather quickly, alcohol took over her life. In fact, by her report, drinking was her life. From her late 20s until she stopped drinking, she spent as much time in various treatment programs as out of them. She can't remember how many times she was in the hospital for detoxification, but guesses it must be at least 50. When Suzie drank, she would often become suicidal, and on numerous occasions, she was admitted to a psychiatric hospital to keep her safe. Suzie became known as a "frequent flyer" because of the number of times she was admitted to the hospital. Both Suzie and the staff came to believe that she probably would never stop drinking.

But Suzie did finally stop drinking. During one admission (her last), she made the decision that she had to change her life. After her detoxification, she went into a longer-term residential program, graduated from it, and never returned to drinking. In fact, Suzie now works in a residential treatment program for people who struggle with substance abuse.

Through my work, I met Suzie and learned of her history of alcohol problems. I was very interested in how she had been able to stop drinking after years of being unable to. What finally did it for her? Was it a counselor she saw, the residential treatment program she got involved in? Maybe it was AA? Did something happen in that last admission that seemed to turn her around? I asked her this, and after thinking a long time, all she could say was, "I guess I was finally ready."

THERE ARE NO MAGIC BULLETS!

A treatment program will not end your problem with alcohol consumption. It is you who must make the decision and make the change. While treatment is often critical for those who need addi-tional help and support, for many people treatment is almost the least important variable. As the saying goes, "you can lead a horse to water, but you can't make it drink." Well, you can force a person into treatment, but unless the person is ready to do something about the problem, treatment will generally not be successful. And this is not a put-down to treatment. While treatment can sometimes help to in-crease a person's motivation to change, be a catalyst for a person to begin a change effort, and provide a chance for an individual to see what life is like without being under the influence of alcohol, it can only do so much. The point is that treatment is no magic bullet. *You are the key and most important ingredient!*

A lot of research has tried to understand what is responsible for successful behavior change when a person sees a therapist, regardless of the type of problem the person is struggling with. What makes treatment work and what is responsible for treatment going well? It should be no surprise to you that, regardless of the specific problem, the most important factor when a person tries to change is the per-son, him- or herself. While having a good social support network is very important, your readiness, motivation, and acceptance of per-sonal responsibility to change are essential.

THE RIGHT ATTITUDE

Again, if you do not have serious psychiatric or other problems, you may be able to help yourself without professional help or attendance at group support meetings. What will help? Some former problem drinkers who resolved their problem report that they had "the right attitude," or that they were ready. However, to say that all it takes is the right attitude and a readiness to change isn't particularly helpful. Many problem drinkers truly want to quit, but for one reason or another have failed over and over again. So what makes it work when it works?

There is one thing we know. You can definitely succeed at resolving your drinking habit even if you have failed before.

Maintaining the Right Attitude

To achieve success, you need to maintain a good attitude. Otherwise there is no way you will be able to cope with the ups and downs you experience as you try to limit alcohol in your life. The right attitude consists of

- *making an intense commitment to change your life.* You need to realize that gaining control over your alcohol consumption is something that you have to do. Changing your relationship to alcohol must become a major life priority. Take responsibility for your drinking and remain committed to changing your use of alcohol.

- *remembering the problems that drinking has caused you (and will cause you) and no longer wanting to deal with those problems.* Without wallowing in the pain related to your past drinking, maintain a clear understanding of the harm you will again experience if you lapse into your old ways. Make the decision to change your pattern of drinking so you will never experience this pain again.

- *finding joy in your life without excessive drinking and never wanting to lose that happiness.* You must work hard to enjoy your life without alcohol. Learn to enjoy life every bit as much, if not more, despite drinking less or not at all. And remember that if you return to uncontrolled drinking, you will lose that happiness and your life will be worse.

- *learning to cope with problems without using alcohol.* Even though you may often feel like drinking, you must deal with your problems without drinking or without drinking excessively. No matter what, drinking to cope can't be an option.

In other words, while you may need to develop new skills and habits, your attitude is more critical than a treatment program. *It will be up to you.* With these four key attitudes, along with the development of certain skills, you will be able to achieve success.

IF PEOPLE CAN HELP THEMSELVES, WHY IS THERE OUTSIDE HELP?

If people can help themselves with their drinking problem, why are professional treatment and self-help groups available? Treatment programs exist because some people find that despite their best efforts, long-term success does not happen without outside help. Some people require objective, professional input. As was previously mentioned, this is particularly true for people who experience other serious difficulties in addition to their drinking problem. Such people may require intensive structure, safe housing, and significant support in order be successful. Even others may not have a social support system to help them with their drinking problem. They may have experienced a number of losses in their lives due to their drinking and the opportunity to obtain other external support is absolutely essential for them to achieve success. Without treatment, some people would not achieve success and would suffer severe consequences as a result of their drinking, including death.

Secondly, some people find it helpful to talk things over with someone who will keep their confidence, who is nonjudgmental, who has their best interests at heart, and who can help them to sort through choices and unseen obstacles. Many people find invaluable support by attending AA, other group meetings, or speaking with a professional therapist.

When you think about it, this same principle operates in other areas. To lose weight, some people want or need to involve themselves in a group program, with weekly meetings and lots of structure. Others may require only a specified diet, which they hold to faithfully. Still others go it alone by watching what they eat and changing their eating habits. As another example, let's take exercise. Some need to join a health club to institute their exercise program. Others will do group aerobics, while some will take up swimming. Others may be able to structure their exercise regimen with exercise equipment in their homes or by jogging. Very simply, different people need, want, and require different input to change their lives. There is no right or wrong road to success, just different routes.

But whatever route a person takes, the most important element is the person's commitment and willingness to change.

◻ ◻ ◻

If you are going to change your relationship to alcohol, it is mostly up to you. You need to make the decision to change your life and stay focused on your goal of getting a handle on your drinking so that you and your loved ones no longer need to suffer from the harm of your drinking. No treatment program can give you that, and it is the most important ingredient to your success. And I believe this is great news, because it means that you have the power and ability to change your use of alcohol.

Along with this determination, you need to work hard to enjoy your life and to learn to cope with stresses, demands, and pressures without drinking. If you have or can develop the necessary beliefs and skills, you will be able to help yourself with your drinking problem. This book is designed to help you to develop these skills.

On the other hand, if you experience uncontrollable emotional stress or severe depression, or you want the support of a therapist or support group, you will do better to seek some additional help and support at the outset. A major point to remember, though, is that whether you seek outside help or decide to tackle your drinking problem on your own, your success will be largely up to you. Your attitude, commitment, and hard work are essential.

5

YOU MAY NEED
MEDICAL HELP

Intelligence is knowing when you need to ask for help.
ANONYMOUS

Even people with severe alcohol problems do not always drink every day. As a result, they may not notice any withdrawal symptoms (described below) even though their bodies may experience some toxicity as a result of their drinking. Usually, such individuals can safely stop drinking without the need for outside medical assistance. For daily drinkers who consume large quantities of alcohol, however, the need for medically assisted detoxification is probably a necessity. If your body has become very used to alcohol, it will be extremely dangerous for you to suddenly stop drinking without medical assistance.

ARE YOU PHYSIOLOGICALLY DEPENDENT UPON ALCOHOL?

The big question: how strongly does your body need alcohol? Without alcohol, do you experience serious bodily stress? If your system has become accustomed to alcohol, your sudden stopping may cause serious and dangerous withdrawal symptoms:

- high blood pressure
- anxiety and tremors
- seizures
- rapid heartbeat
- increased sweating
- auditory, visual, and tactile hallucinations
- delirium
- mental confusion and agitation
- nausea and vomiting
- headache
- inability to sleep

In many cases these symptoms are few and relatively mild. In other cases, they can be so severe as to cause further damage to your system. If you suffer any of these symptoms—even if slight—when you stop consuming alcohol, you need to consult a medical professional. If you need some alcohol in the morning to "stop the shakes," you require detoxification.

Severe alcohol problems need medically supervised detoxification. If you are subject to withdrawal symptoms, medical detoxification involves replacing the alcohol in your system with another drug. This will allow you to withdraw from alcohol gradually and safely— usually over a four- or five-day period. Who will experience alcohol withdrawal symptoms? Generally, the risk of withdrawal is greater

— the more people drink, especially if they drink heavily daily;
— the more years a person has been drinking;

— for older drinkers; and

— for people who have experienced withdrawal problems in the past, even if long ago.

DRINKING CAN CAUSE OTHER MEDICAL PROBLEMS

In addition to alcohol withdrawal problems, the heavy regular use of alcohol can cause other damage for which you may need to see your doctor:

- anemia
- gastrointestinal bleeding
- liver disease
- pancreatitis
- alcoholic myopathy
- congestive heart failure
- dehydration
- cognitive and memory impairment

Any of these medical conditions may abate with abstinence, but they also can become permanent. Consequently, if you have been drinking a lot, it would be a good idea to have your doctor examine you in order to ensure that your medical condition is stable and that you do not have any serious health problem that requires intervention and treatment.

The safest and best advice is to see a medical doctor. It can't hurt, and you can rule out any medical problems. You will then do what is best for your health.

MEDICAL DETOXIFICATION: WHAT HAPPENS

The most common setting for medical detoxification is an inpatient hospital program. There you will be given medication to prevent an acute, sudden, and potentially dangerous withdrawal syndrome. Large amounts of this medication will be given to start with and then gradually tapered over the course of four or five days. This will allow your body to get used to not having alcohol in your system without placing undue stress on your physical or emotional health. During your hospitalization, you will also receive individual and group counseling to help you to remain alcohol-free. Family members may also be asked to participate in your treatment.

THE TIMES ARE A-CHANGING

Significant changes have occurred and continue to take place in the treatment of alcohol problems during the past 20 years. In fact, our entire health care system, including the treatment of medical and mental illnesses, has changed during this time. The primary reason for this shift is the financial costs of health care and the need to reduce these costs.

Inpatient hospital care is very expensive, with a one-day charge ranging from several hundred dollars to over one thousand dollars, depending upon the type of care that is required. As a result, many researchers have examined whether people need to be in a hospital to receive the care they need. The length of time that people need to be in the hospital has also been reevaluated.

Regarding the treatment of alcohol problems, 15 to 20 years ago it was very common for a person to be admitted to a hospital for detoxification and then to remain in the hospital for an additional three weeks for extended rehabilitation, which was all covered by health insurance. The 28-day program was the standard treatment for an alcohol problem. Because of the enormous cost of a hospital stay of this length, however, insurance companies and researchers began to study whether this was necessary.

Essentially, they found that people who stayed in the hospital for 28 days did no better than those who spent a much shorter time in the hospital and then participated in structured outpatient treatment. As a result, nowadays, if a person needs to go into a hospital for detoxification, most likely insurance will pay only for several days there, just long enough for medical detoxification. The person is then discharged and referred to other community supports.

There are, though, still some 28-day programs available. Some are state-supported public programs, and others must be paid for out-of-pocket unless your health insurance covers this cost. These types of programs are discussed in chapter 16.

DETOXIFYING WHILE LIVING AT HOME

Some people today go through medical detoxification on an outpatient basis without ever being in the hospital. Again, as a way to save money, it was reasoned that people could be safely detoxified while living at home and receive the same or similar individual and group counseling on an outpatient basis that they would receive in a hospital. This type of outpatient detoxification makes sense for those who are reasonably physically and emotionally healthy, who have never had and are not in danger of having a severe alcohol withdrawal syndrome, and who have adequate social support in their homes. A doctor can determine whether this is safe for you. While you are being detoxified and receiving tapering doses of medication, you will also receive counseling to help you to decide upon any aftercare treatment that you may need. This is likely to involve an outpatient substance abuse treatment program.

Detoxification, however, is only the first step. Learning how to stop alcohol from ruining your life is the next objective.

6

WHAT TO DO:
ABSTINENCE OR MODERATION?

People are usually more convinced by reasons they dis-
covered themselves than by those found by others.

BLAISE PASCAL

Okay, you are now ready to stop alcohol from hurting your life. In order to do this, you need to change your relationship with alcohol. You are probably wondering if you should try to moderate your drinking or if you need to stop drinking entirely. This chapter will help you to make that decision.

As a first choice, most people prefer to control alcohol intake so that it stops causing problems in their lives. At least at some point, most people who drink too much have entertained this desire. They want to continue to drink and have that pleasure, but without all of the problems that formerly went with it. They want to be like other people who drink safely and without doing themselves or others harm. Non-problem drinkers seldom, if ever, drink to excess, they generally do not become seriously intoxicated, and overall, alcohol does not interfere in their lives. Very simply, no problems result from their moderate alcohol consumption. One way of ending many of your problems may be to learn how to drink in moderation.

TRYING TO MODERATE DRINKING IS CONTROVERSIAL . . .

As I discussed in chapter 2, many people and professional organizations maintain that a drinking problem is a disease and that the best, if not only, way to recover from a drinking problem is by completely abstaining from alcohol. Alcoholics Anonymous also believes that abstinence is the only way to recover from a drinking problem. Remember that from the point of view that an alcohol problem is a disease, any drinking will eventually escalate to more drinking because the "loss-of-control" phenomenon is real and a part of the illness. It is thought that it is simply impossible for an alcoholic to moderate drinking, and in truth, many people who drink too much can't control their drinking. One drink leads to way too many.

YET SOME PEOPLE CAN DO IT

As I also discussed in chapter 2, in contrast to the disease perspective, a drinking problem can be more like a bad habit. This perspective opens the door to the possibility that a person can learn to drink differently. Many people who have experienced a problem with alcohol have learned to change their destructive pattern of drinking. So, although the technique of moderating drinking is controversial, it is clearly a possibility for some people.

HOW COMMON IS MODERATE DRINKING?

Reports of individuals learning how to control their drinking after first having had problems with drinking vary from study to study. Some studies report that only about 5 percent of people who have experienced a drinking problem can learn to moderate their drinking. Not very good odds. Yet other studies report that 30 percent or even 60 percent of people who have had a drinking problem can learn moderation. Obviously, much better odds. Why the huge range?

My own practice mirrors these findings. I sometimes find that three or even four out of five people who want to control their drinking are able to. But at another time, I might find that only one out of five can do this, or maybe no one can. Again, why the range and what is responsible for this? The wide range in successful moderate drinking observed in studies is due to several factors, including how long ago people first experienced an alcohol problem, how controlled drinking is defined, and, most important, who is actually studied.

In general, the longer ago people first experienced an alcohol problem, the more reports of people controlling their drinking are found. The same is true for abstinence-oriented outcomes because, over time, people with alcohol problems get better either via abstinence or by learning to moderate their drinking. When people who report that they recently experienced a problem with alcohol are studied, the percentage of people who are moderating their drinking is less than among people who report that they first experienced an alcohol problem a long time ago. How controlled drinking is defined is also important. Obviously, with a very conservative definition, there will be fewer reports of controlled drinking, whereas with a somewhat more liberal definition, the numbers of people who moderate their drinking will be greater.

Finally and most important is the type of people who are being studied, which can greatly affect the observed rates of successful controlled drinking. Individuals with more severe alcohol problems seem to do best with an abstinence-oriented approach, whereas those with less severe problems are more able to learn how to moderate their drinking. Based upon the severity of alcohol problems among the people who are being studied, rates of controlled drinking will greatly vary. Some people have a very good probability of learning how to moderate their drinking, whereas others have a much smaller chance.

Related to the severity of the alcohol problem is the fact that rates of controlled drinking are also greater for individuals who never received treatment for their alcohol problem. In general, people who seek treatment for a drinking problem have more significant problems related to alcohol than those who have not received treatment. Typically, an alcohol problem goes on for many years before a person is willing to seek and get involved in treatment. Treatment is often avoided until there is outside pressure to do this, and often the pressure results from consistent and severe problems related to alcohol consumption. As a result, if a study looks only at people who received treatment, the rates of controlled drinking will be less. Furthermore, because most treatment programs focus exclusively on abstinence as the only route to recovery, those who have received treatment may tend to choose this path to resolve their problem as opposed to individuals who have helped themselves without treatment. In turn, rates of controlled drinking among individuals who have received treatment will be less. So what are your chances of learning to moderate your drinking?

IT DEPENDS ON THE PERSON

The truth of the matter is that there is such a big range because it depends on who the person is and the type of drinking problem he has. Drinking problems vary in severity and type, so some people have a very good probability of learning how to moderate their drinking, whereas others have a much smaller chance. So what are your chances of learning to moderate your drinking?

WHO CAN MODERATE THEIR DRINKING?

You'll have the best chance of learning how to moderate your drinking if these conditions apply to you:

- You have never been physically dependent upon alcohol (have never experienced the alcohol withdrawal syndrome described in chapter 5).
- You are not a daily drinker.
- You have had a drinking problem for less than 10 years. Think about your history of drinking. You may have started drinking a long time ago, but have you had a drinking *problem* for a long time?
- You have not had severe problems related to drinking. Think long and hard about the effect alcohol has had on your life. Has drinking caused you severe problems like loss of jobs and relationships, legal problems, or other major hardships?
- You have had past periods of successfully not drinking or of moderating your drinking.
- You are employed. Employment structures your day and improves your chances of successful moderate drinking.
- You are psychologically stable. Is drinking your main problem or do you struggle with other emotional concerns such as significant depression or anxiety?
- You have friends and family who are not heavy drinkers.

- You are under age 40. (Age matters because it correlates with number of years of drinking.)
- You very much want to moderate your drinking.
- You have a social environment that supports moderate drinking. Not only is it important that the people around you aren't heavy drinkers, but you need people around you who support your wish to moderate your drinking.

Before you try this approach, if you are taking any prescribed medication, you should check with your doctor first to see if you can drink while taking your medication. And if you are pregnant, you should not drink at all as alcohol can have harmful effects on your fetus. A good recommendation before attempting controlled drinking is to get a physical exam by your doctor to confirm that it is not a medical problem for you to drink.

WHO SHOULD CHOOSE ABSTINENCE?

You'll do best with an abstinence-oriented approach if the following conditions apply to you:

- You have had a drinking problem for more than 10 years. Take a good look at your drinking history and the effect alcohol has had on your life. If your misuse of alcohol has been going on for many years, you'll do best by stopping drinking entirely.
- You drink every day, or just about every day, and rarely have days when you do not drink.
- You have experienced many problems due to your drinking. Again, take a long and hard look at the influence alcohol has

had on your life. Has it caused you many problems, whether this consists of loss of jobs, broken relationships, legal difficulties, or financial problems?

- You have been or are physically dependent upon alcohol. When you stop drinking, do you experience the alcohol withdrawal syndrome described in chapter 5?
- You have been told by your doctor not to drink.
- You have previously tried to moderate your drinking with only limited success.
- You are surrounded by heavy drinkers. If your social network, including friends and family, are into the heavy drinking scene, the chances are that you will need to abstain from alcohol to prevent it from hurting your life.

Many people intuitively know whether they will need to completely abstain from alcohol to recover from their alcohol problem. From their history, they know for themselves that one drink inevitably has led to too many and that total abstinence will be the only way to avoid this. They may have tried numerous times to control their drinking without success. If this sounds familiar to you, I would suggest the route of abstinence.

ABSTINENCE OR MODERATION?

Perhaps you've read my recommendations, and even though you don't fit the description of someone who is likely to be able to control drinking through moderation, you still want to try to see if you can learn to control it. You think that with effort, you may be able to achieve success. Who knows, you *may* be right! There are people who have had severe problems with alcohol who, much to my surprise, beat the odds.

This book is about your taking control of how you want to address your problem with alcohol. While the chances are against your being able to learn to drink in moderation, you may still want to try. You may feel that you first need to see whether you can do this before you consider abstinence. If this is what you want to do, go for it. However, again, if this is your plan, first check with your doctor to make sure that it is okay for you to drink at all.

ONE CAVEAT

Some of you may have resolved your alcohol problem by not drinking at all. If abstinence is working for you, great. Don't change a thing. As the saying goes, "If it's not broken, don't fix it." Stay the course if it's working.

⬜ ⬜ ⬜

In this chapter, I have explained what type of drinker has the best chance of resolving a drinking problem by learning how to moderate it and what type should choose the path of abstinence. Now is the time for you to think long and hard about which category you fit into. Reread my recommendations and take an honest look at yourself and your relationship to alcohol. Decide which category most describes you and commit to a course of action. Now is the time to stop alcohol from ruining your life and to start feeling better about yourself. No matter what your decision, the very fact that you recognize you have a problem is something to be proud of.

The next part of this book is devoted to strategies to help you moderate your drinking. If your decision is to abstain, skip to part IV. Either of these paths can help; you just need to follow the correct one for you. Good luck—but it really takes more than luck. It takes a commitment to change your life and hard work. If you keep this in mind, you will succeed.

PART III

MODERATING YOUR DRINKING

7

MODERATION:
GENERAL TECHNIQUES

To enjoy freedom we have to control ourselves.
VIRGINIA WOOLF

Moderation means being able to control or limit your drinking to a level that does not interfere in your life. Your goal is to learn to drink in a way so that drinking does not cause you financial, vocational, physical, legal, emotional, or social difficulties, or any other problems. To accomplish this, the amount of alcohol that you consume must be within reasonable limits and less than what you used to drink. There are many techniques to help you moderate your drinking. These techniques must be the backdrop and foundation of the individualized moderate drinking contract you will develop in the next chapter.

SIP AND ENJOY YOUR DRINKS

Sipping your drinks will greatly slow down your drinking and make it easier for you to moderate your alcohol intake. Try putting your drink on the table or bar between sips. This will slow you down because continuing to hold your drink leads to more rapid drinking. If the drink remains in your hand, it's easy to drink it quickly. You'll be surprised at how long you can make a drink last and how much you will still enjoy drinking. One way to make this transition easier is to play a game with yourself to see how slowly you can finish a drink.

Another suggestion is to focus on the flavor of the drink. Typically, people who drink too much chug their drinks and don't even taste what they are drinking. They drink to get drunk, which is exactly what you do not want to do. You need to focus on the taste rather than on getting drunk.

DON'T DRINK SHOTS, MULTI-SHOT DRINKS, OR PUNCHES

In light of what I just said, it makes sense that you should stay away from drinking shots of hard liquor, because it is hard to make a shot last a long time. Drinking shots is an easy way to drink too quickly and too much.

You should also stay away from multi-shot drinks such as martinis, Rob Roys, or Black Russians. These have more alcohol content in them than single-shot mixed drinks and do not qualify as just *one* drink. They are much stronger and tend to be drunk too quickly as well.

Punches are also dangerous because you don't always know what type of alcohol is in them or how strong they are. You may think that you are having only one drink, but in reality, the alcohol content may equal two or more drinks. They are also very easy to chug or drink quickly, especially if you're thirsty.

DON'T DRINK WHEN YOU'RE THIRSTY

When people are thirsty, they automatically drink fluid to relieve their thirst. If you drink alcohol when you are thirsty, you will tend to drink more quickly and in all probability you will have a tendency to drink more. Alcohol, too, can actually make you thirstier because it dehydrates you. Drinking alcohol causes you to sweat, increases the production of urine, and results in a loss of body water. So when you drink to quench your thirst, it has the opposite effect. When you are thirsty, the best thing is to drink water. Have a glass or two of water to first quench your thirst before drinking any alcohol.

EAT WHEN YOU DRINK

Eat when you drink, and never drink on an empty stomach. Having food in your stomach will slow down the rate at which alcohol gets into your bloodstream. This will help to diminish the effects of alcohol and will prevent rapid intoxication that can lead you to make poorer decisions about your drinking. One note of caution, though: don't eat salty foods, which increase your thirst and lead to more drinking. Stay away from the peanuts, chips, fries, and other salty snacks.

HAVE ONLY A LIMITED SUPPLY OF ALCOHOL AT HOME

If you drink mostly when you are at home, you shouldn't have a lot of alcohol on hand. Having alcohol readily accessible can make drinking, and over-drinking, way too tempting. Limiting the amount of alcohol you keep around your home will help you to moderate your drinking.

PREPARE YOUR MINDSET

When you plan to drink or know that you will be in a drinking situation, you need to actively remind yourself that you are trying to limit your drinking. You need to prepare yourself in advance and enter these situations with a focused and determined mindset. In the next chapter, you will learn to create your individualized moderate drinking contract, which will ensure that your drinking stays within safe limits. Once you have developed this, before going to any social situation, think about your contract and be determined to follow it.

DELAY HAVING YOUR FIRST ALCOHOLIC DRINK

When you first enter a drinking situation, wait to have your first alcoholic drink. Give yourself time to adjust to and enjoy the setting without using alcohol. After you are already enjoying yourself, have a drink if you want. This will help to get you in the right frame of mind—the one in which you keep a watchful eye on your drinking. If you really need to have a drink in your hand to feel at ease, make it one without alcohol.

STAY FOCUSED ON MODERATION

In a social situation where everyone is drinking, you need to stay focused and not allow yourself to get caught up in the camaraderie of heavy drinking. For example, when a group of people are out to dinner, it is very common when one person orders another drink for everyone else to follow suit without thinking too much about whether they really want another. Or, if a person is buying a drink for himself, he may offer to buy drinks for others, and again, without thinking much about it, everyone jumps on the bandwagon. You need to be mindful of this scenario.

GET PLEASURE FROM THE SOCIAL SITUATION

When in a social situation, even though drinking may be a part of the scene, there is much more to do than drink. You can meet new people, reconnect with old friends, listen to music, etc. Whether you are playing softball, swimming, dancing, or playing cards, you can keep the focus on controlling your drinking while getting your enjoyment from everything else going on around you. If you can center your energy on all the other pleasurable aspects of the situation, you'll naturally place less emphasis on drinking. You may find that you enjoy these things more now that you are concentrating less on getting drunk.

LET'S GET STARTED

The best way to begin your new life of moderation is to take a two-week break from drinking before you start to try to control your drinking. If that sounds too long, try to go at least one week without alcohol. This exercise is helpful for a number of reasons.

First, with moderate drinking, I strongly recommend that you do not drink every day. I know this can be a challenge if you are used to drinking most every day. But relax, you can do this. You need to get used to not drinking, and taking a one- or two-week break will strengthen your confidence in your ability to not drink. This will be very useful once you actually start your plan to moderate your drinking.

Second, for many of you, moderate drinking will be a lifestyle change. You will be drinking less and less often than you presently do, and you may need to find other things to do with your time. During this fairly brief period of not drinking, experiment with new hobbies or spend more time on those you have always enjoyed. Filling your time with rewarding activities will be valuable in keeping alcohol from being a major part of your life forever.

There may be certain times when you miss drinking or when you feel like drinking more than at other times. Again, not drinking will build your confidence and let you know that despite wanting to drink, you can choose not to. Also, discovering when you really want to drink can give you insight into the role alcohol plays in your life and what you need to better manage without it. For example, if you feel like drinking after a stressful day at work, you will need to find other ways to relax after a long day. Or if you feel like drinking more when you feel angry or upset, you can work on learning to cope with these feelings in other ways.

MODERATING YOUR DRINKING ISN'T SOCIAL DRINKING

A social drinker does not think about when to drink, how to drink, how much to drink, or what type of alcohol to drink. A social drinker does not need to prepare his mindset and doesn't worry about getting drunk or the possibility that drinking can get out of control and cause problems. For social drinkers, alcohol is simply not an issue: they can take it or leave it.

For someone who is moderating her drinking, drinking is an issue and needs to be thought about seriously. Moderate drinkers must *always* remain vigilant and mindful of how much they drink because the possibility of drinking too much remains very real. They must also remember all of the mental attitudes that will enable successful moderate drinking: a strong commitment to change, awareness of the harmful consequences of excessive alcohol consumption, finding joy in life without drinking and not wanting to lose that, and being able to deal with life stress and internal urges without turning to alcohol. Let's now look at the specific elements of the moderate drinking contract by which you will learn to live.

8

YOUR PERSONAL
MODERATE DRINKING CONTRACT

*Unless commitment is made, there are only promises
and hopes; but no plans.*   PETER F. DRUCKER

To learn to moderate your drinking and to make it as easy as possible,
you need to make a contract with yourself that clearly outlines how
much, how often, and when and where you can drink. You can't
simply "cut down" or make a conscious decision to drink less. This
contract with yourself symbolizes your *total commitment to yourself* to
get your drinking under control and will specify clear rules for you to
live and drink by.

WHY ARE CLEAR RULES IMPORTANT?

Rules give you structure, which is essential because your drinking has
been out of control. Laying out clear drinking rules gives you the firm
guidelines you need to bring your drinking into control. As your
drinking has had no boundaries or controls, you need structure to

contain your drinking. Safe drinking rules that you agree to follow provide explicit targets and goals and a clear path to pursue to limit your drinking. Without such rules, chances are you won't get a handle on your drinking.

Developing firm rules that you agree to consistently follow is also a good way for you to know whether or not you can truly moderate your drinking . . . *not some of the time, but all of the time*. If you cannot abide by the rules of moderate drinking you establish, it means that you can't moderate your drinking and that abstinence is the better route for you.

Creating clear rules will prevent your slipping back to old habits. For example, let's assume that you used to drink two six-packs of beer and have decided to "cut down," without setting a clear rule. Then you control your drinking so that you sometimes drink four beers, other days you drink six, and over time, your drinking increases and you sometimes drink eight or ten. While you have "cut down," is this truly moderating your drinking? Clearly not. Developing clear limits on how much you can and will safely drink—*all of the time*—will keep you on track and prevent your drinking from escalating.

THE SIX CRUCIAL QUESTIONS OF YOUR MODERATE DRINKING CONTRACT

In this chapter, you'll learn to outline the specifics of your moderate drinking contract by answering six crucial questions. Before you fill out the contract that appears at the end of this chapter, you'll have to clearly understand each of these elements that will allow you to succeed. This contract will be the document you will live by as you learn to moderate your drinking.

1. How Much Can You Drink?

The first question you need to answer is how many drinks you can safely consume in one sitting. I believe that a maximum of three standard drinks is more than enough for any person. Three drinks is the upper limit because this amount is not enough to greatly intoxicate most people. (Of course, if you become intoxicated by three drinks, your personal limit should be lower.) When you drink more than this amount, your judgment can become impaired, making it difficult to exercise good decision making. Adhering to this limit is crucial to complying with your drinking contract.

If you are struggling with the three-drink limit, you may increase your limit to four, but I don't recommend this when you are first starting off. Later on, after you have demonstrated good control, it may be possible for you to be somewhat more flexible with this limit. For now, though, stick to a three-drink limit. If you can't be satisfied with three drinks, moderate drinking may not be the best option for you.

When suggesting drinking limits, you should know that the National Institute of Alcohol Abuse and Alcoholism suggests that women drink no more than one drink per day or seven drinks per week and that men should consume a maximum of two drinks per day or 14 drinks per week. The World Health Organization (WHO) has a somewhat more liberal recommendation regarding low-risk drinking: about 3 drinks per day or 21 drinks per week for men and slightly less than 2 drinks each day or about 14 drinks per week for women. Men who drink 5 or more drinks in a day or more than 15 in a week, and women who drink 4 or more in a day or 8 in one week have an increased risk of developing alcohol-related problems.

These are general guidelines and everyone is different. A person's metabolism, age, weight, and medical status can greatly affect how alcohol interacts with that person's body. So I strongly recommend that you speak with your physician about what should be your limit when deciding how many drinks you should have in one sitting.

As I just mentioned, weight is a factor as heavier people generally can handle more alcohol than those who weigh less. So when thinking about your limit, take this into account and, if you weigh less than the average woman or man, go with a smaller limit.

You should also know that, for some people, four drinks, or even three, may be too many because this can easily turn into drinking five or six. In this circumstance, you may think of limiting yourself to a maximum of one or two.

What Is a Drink? When suggesting guidelines about how much you can drink, we need to talk about what is meant by "a drink." A standard drink is equivalent to a 12-ounce bottle of beer, five ounces of wine, or one-and-a-half ounces of eighty-proof hard liquor. These are "honest," measured drinks, and not the tumbler-size ones you might have occasionally consumed. When pouring drinks, you will need to start measuring them, at least initially. Once you get more used to these amounts, you may be able to gauge them without measuring. But no cheating, as you will only be kidding yourself.

Women Are Different from Men. As I just noted, recommendations put forth by leading agencies regarding low-risk drinking guidelines consistently suggest lower limits for women as compared to men. Women have a higher proportion of fat in their bodies in relation to water and tend to feel the effects of alcohol more than do men. This is why I agree with the guidelines that suggest lowering the limits for women as compared to men. For women, keeping to a three-drink limit, or even two, is strongly recommended because of physiology.

You Can Drink Less but Never More! Just because your upper limit is three doesn't mean you must *always* drink this amount. In fact, a good sign of being able to control your drinking is that you are able to choose to have one or two on some days. This doesn't mean you can go over your limit on other days!

Slow Down, and Don't Gulp Your Drinks. Consume only one drink per hour. This prevents intoxication and will decrease the chances of your having alcohol-related problems. Looking at a clock and pacing drinking is critical to your success. Sipping your drink, putting your drink down, and focusing on the taste will help you to do this (review chapter 7).

Don't Forget about Non-alcoholic Drinks. It is useful to intersperse non-alcoholic drinks with alcoholic ones, especially in social situations where you are used to having a drink in your hands. Non-alcoholic drinks include water or sparkling water, soda, fruit juices, or even non-alcoholic beer or wine. There is certainly nothing wrong with holding and drinking any type of these non-alcoholic drinks. Have as many as you like. Drinking in this fashion will help to keep your alcohol consumption in control.

Start Off with a Non-alcoholic Drink. Particularly useful when in social situations, start off with a non-alcoholic drink first. Your mindset is key (see chapter 7). If you know that you are going to be somewhere for a long time and drinking is a part of the scene, starting with an alcohol-free beverage will help to focus on limiting your drinking and keeping it in control. Your mindset will be on moderating your drinking and not on getting drunk.

Kathy usually drank without any problems, except on the weekends when socializing and drinking with a group of friends. In that setting, she would often over-drink, which was beginning to cause problems between her and her husband. She also didn't like how she felt the next day. Her trick was to begin the evening with one or two non-alcoholic drinks, which would delay the start time of her drinking. She learned that doing this set the stage for her entire evening—instead of jumping into the evening with alcohol in order to feel its effects, this delay helped her to remain focused on moderating her drinking, and she enjoyed the evening while having only two or three alcoholic drinks.

Make Sure to Eat. Not only is it a good idea to eat food when you drink, it's an even better idea to eat something *before* drinking. Having food in your stomach slows the rate at which alcohol enters your system. This, in turn, decreases the effect alcohol has on you and makes it easier to adhere to your drinking limits.

2. What Can You Drink?

While typically "a drink is a drink is a drink," and all alcoholic drinks have the capacity to cause you to lose control, it is possible that certain kinds of alcohol may cause you more problems than others. For example, some people can drink beer without a problem, but if they drink hard liquor, even when diluted, it's another story. Others find they can maintain control by sticking to wine. In fact, unless diluted, hard liquor, with its greater percentage of alcohol, gets into your system more quickly than does a drink with a lower percentage of alcohol such as beer or wine. So, remember, it is harder to maintain control if you drink hard liquor. Limiting alcohol consumption to only beer or wine will help you to maintain control.

Just as you can alternate alcoholic beverages with non-alcoholic ones to help limit your drinking, if you still want to be able to drink hard liquor, it may also work for you to dilute your hard liquor with a greater amount of mixer. Drinking this way helps to make the drinks last much longer and will help to keep your drinking in control.

Switching to a less preferred alcoholic beverage can also help to control drinking. For example, if wine is your favorite beverage and what you always drink, changing to beer can help you to drink less.

If you are an individual who runs into problems no matter what you drink, or you start off with a less preferred beverage but soon go back to your favorite, problematic one, you need to remain abstinent to resolve your drinking problem. For you, "a drink is a drink is a drink."

3. How Often Can You Drink?

A good guideline is to drink three or at most four days per week. Of course, drinking less is always a good choice.

The Four-Day Limit. Drinking more than four days per week is dangerous because drinking can escalate to daily drinking, which increases your chances of repeating alcohol-related problems. If you can't imagine having some days on which you do not drink, then moderate drinking is not for you and you should choose total abstinence.

Second, having three days every week without alcohol helps you prevent developing a tolerance to alcohol. Tolerance is when your body gets used to alcohol and more alcohol is needed to feel an effect. Remember back to when one drink used to make you feel relaxed? Over time, you probably needed two drinks to create the same feeling, then three or even four. Abstinent days are very important in helping you to moderate your drinking.

Finally, having non-drinking days forces you to do other things with your life that do not include or revolve around drinking. This is key, since moderate drinking demands you change your lifestyle. Having other activities that you enjoy doing makes moderating your drinking much easier. For example, instead of your usual pattern of going home after work and drinking, go to the health club, go shopping, see a movie, enroll in a class, or meet some friends for coffee. Or if you go home, change your usual routine and go for a walk or jog, read a book, involve yourself in a house project, or develop some other leisure activity.

4. When Can You Drink . . . and 5. When Can't You Drink?

Your next step is to establish the types of situations in which you can drink and, equally as important, the types of situations in which you should avoid drinking. Over the course of your life, you, like everyone who drinks, have developed a drinking pattern. There are times or situations when your drinking is generally in control and you only have a few drinks. There are also times when your drinking has been excessive. If you are going to successfully control your drinking, you need to analyze your drinking pattern to pinpoint your "low-risk" and "high-risk" situations.

"Low risk" means those situations you are in, or people you are with, when you have been able to drink safely and in control. "High risk" means the places, times, or people that cause you to drink too much. So you need to identify those specific situations that are low risk for you and make a rule to only drink in those situations. You also need to identify your high-risk situations and to make a rule to never drink when in those.

Al, a successful 38-year-old father of two children, discovered that he would never over-drink when he drank at home while his family was around. However, when he stopped off at the local tavern after work with some of his coworkers, he would generally drink too much and would arrive home late, and problems would ensue between him and his wife. One of his rules was only to drink when home with his family and to never drink at the tavern.

Charlie, 29 years old and single, realized that with certain friends who were not heavy drinkers he would never lose control of his drinking. However, with another group, his friends from high school who drank heavily, he would often drink too much. To moderate his drinking, he made the rule not to drink with his high school friends and to see them less.

Times of the Day. There may be particular times during your daily routine when you tend to slip in a drink or two, which then often leads to more. If there are, make the rule not to drink during those times. Mary, a 32-year-old married woman, realized that if she began to drink while preparing dinner for her family, she would often drink too much. However, if she waited until she sat down with her family for dinner to have her first drink, she would not over-drink and her drinking was much easier to control. Bob discovered that if he first started to drink at home before going out to a bar, he would drink too much. However, if he waited to have his first drink at the bar, he could control his drinking.

Your State of Mind. While a person can always find a reason to drink, there may be certain psychological states that have tended to trigger your heavier drinking. For example, painful emotional states—anger, loneliness, sadness, stress, or frustration—are often triggers.

Think about whether there are feelings that have historically spurred your drinking. What are they? Once you list them, make the decision not to drink when feeling that way. Obviously, you will need to develop other ways to manage your feelings, especially the painful ones. You should think of more constructive things to do and healthier ways to cope when you are feeling bad. Talking with a friend, taking a warm bath, going for a jog, listening to music, reading a book, or meditating are just a few examples of other things you can do to cope with some difficult feelings.

For example, Wayne noticed that whenever he had a stressful day at work, he liked to relax with a drink before having dinner with his wife. During these times, he often lost control of his drinking. As a way to moderate his alcohol intake, he made a rule never to drink during these times of stress. Instead, he learned other ways to relax, which included meditation, reading, and exercise. He also was surprised to find that sitting down with his wife before dinner with only a club soda and lemon helped him to unwind as well. It was taking the time to relax and talk about his day, rather than the alcohol per se, that did the trick.

6. What Situations Should You Totally Avoid?

Despite your best intentions not to drink when in any of your high-risk situations, you may find that this is simply not possible. For example, most of your friends may be heavy drinkers. You may have decided not to drink when you're with these friends, because your drinking is heavier when you're around them. Even if you resolve not to drink in this situation, in truth it may be very difficult if not impossible. A better rule for you would be to not place yourself in such a situation in the first place.

Several years ago, I worked with Sam, a 43-year-old married man who wanted to learn to control his drinking. In reviewing his drinking with me, Sam realized that whenever he went out to dinner with his wife, he could consistently have one or two drinks and would never over-drink. However, whenever he socialized with a particular set of heavy-drinking friends in group settings, he would regularly drink too much, although he had made a rule to never drink when he saw these friends. He discovered that whenever he socialized with them, he couldn't refrain from drinking (and from drinking too much). He was forced to make the rule to stop seeing these friends in group situations. Fortunately, Sam didn't have to give up these friends entirely. He spoke with them and was able to see them on an individual basis when heavy drinking was not in the picture. He also found that if he went out to dinner with his wife, and one of his friends and his wife joined them, he could moderate his drinking as well.

Tom is a 23-year-old single man who came to me at his lawyer's suggestion. While extremely intoxicated, he was arrested for breaking into a retail store. Although he didn't remember why he broke into the store, he had a vague recollection of the police finding him in the store after the burglar alarm had been set off. Tom was a heavy drinker who would stop off at a bar a couple of times each week and could consume between one and two quarts of gin when he drank. He rarely drank at home and realized that the only time he drank so heavily was when he met his friends at the bar. As a way to control his drinking, he decided that he could only drink at home and never go to the bar, where he knew he would over-drink.

THREE IMPORTANT CONTRACT RULES

So now you have a clear understanding of the six elements you need to outline in your moderate drinking contract. However, before you get started on writing your contract, there are three other rules you need to know.

1. Don't Be Discouraged

Don't be discouraged if your spouse or other family members or your drinking buddies think that your goal of trying to moderate your drinking is ridiculous. They probably have good reason. How often have they heard you say, "I won't drink that much . . . I'll only have a couple," only to watch you proceed to over-drink? Or perhaps you stopped drinking for some time and then started again, leading to your drinking eventually getting out of control.

You need to remember that most people, including your family members, believe that total abstinence is the only way to resolve a drinking problem. They may think that trying to moderate your drinking is simply a fantasy resulting from your unwillingness to admit you have a problem. As a result, family members may think that the whole idea of you trying to moderate your drinking is crazy and doomed to fail. They may feel angry that you are continuing to drink, or at a minimum, they will be confused about what you are doing. The key is not to be discouraged if you firmly believe you are able to moderate your drinking.

Getting Support for a Moderate Drinking Contract. Communicate, communicate, and communicate. Talk with your spouse, family members, or others close to you who have been affected by your drinking. Talk about what you are doing, and after you complete your moderate drinking contract, show it to them and try to enlist their support. Make sure they understand what you are attempting to do so that you will have their backing. Explain to them that their support will help you more than their confusion, resentment, or anger.

Don't simply say to them that you are trying to "cut down" your drinking. How many times have you probably said this to them already? Rather, explain to them that you are trying to moderate your drinking and show them your moderate drinking contract. This will demonstrate how well you have thought this out. You should also let them know that you plan to stop drinking entirely if you can't successfully moderate your drinking. This should ease their concern about what you are attempting to do and help you to gain their support.

I am reminded of Steve, a 46-year-old, very successful businessman, who had been married to Sandy for 14 years. Prior to seeing me, Steve had just been discharged from an inpatient detoxification program after being referred there by his employer. For the previous three years, Steve had been drinking at least five times per week and had consumed one or two pints of gin each night. Steve used to smoke marijuana daily, and when his supply ran out, he turned to alcohol. Steve drank at home after work to relieve tension, and his drinking had greatly affected his relationship with his wife. In fact, Steve and Sandy were sleeping in separate bedrooms, and she was considering a separation. Both of Steve's parents were alcoholic, and he figured that he was as well. He hated the idea of being alcoholic, as this meant that he could not drink, and he still wanted to.

During the next week, Steve remained abstinent, but the following week, he had a few drinks. His wife knew nothing about it. He felt guilty about covering this up and worried that if his wife found out, it would be disastrous for the marriage. Steve wondered if he could learn how to moderate his drinking, as he greatly preferred this over abstinence. Based upon how much Steve used to drink in the past, I had great reservations about whether he could learn moderation. Steve wanted to try, though, and decided that on four evenings each week, he would drink at most three drinks a couple of hours before going to bed. That would be the only time when he would drink. Before implementing this plan, Sandy was invited to our next session, because her blessings and knowledge of Steve's plan were absolutely essential. In fact, without her support, Steve's attempt to moderate his drinking wouldn't have worked. Steve's drinking was such a sore and painful issue that, without Sandy's being fully informed and involved with Steve's plan, any drinking would have caused a huge fight between them.

In that session, although Sandy expressed her concerns, she was grateful that Steve was being honest and open with her. As Sandy learned more about his plan and the specific moderate drinking contract he had developed, she gave Steve her support. Steve adhered to his contract over the next three months, and sometimes he didn't even have all three drinks or drink on all four nights.

The Importance of Friends. Good friends will respect your decision, and their knowing about your plan will decrease the chance that they will offer you a drink or without thinking refill your glass when it is empty. Informing them about your intentions may also decrease the subtle encouragement to drink more and get drunk that often happens among friends in drinking situations. This will make it easier for you to moderate your drinking. The straightforward act of informing others may also help to further your commitment and make it harder for you to violate your contract.

2. Moderate Drinking Rules Are Not to Be Broken

Initially, the rules you make should be followed religiously. Bending and changing them will lead to your drinking getting out of control again. The one exception is to change rules to include *less* drinking or to decrease your chances of over-drinking. As you'll see in the next chapter, you may find that you need additional structure to successfully control your drinking.

Why You Can't Change Your Rules. Until you have demonstrated good control and are successfully moderating your drinking for a period of three months, you should not change your drinking rules. Early temptations to change your rules are likely because you are having difficulty in holding to your contract. This signifies that your drinking is still out of control, and you need to first demonstrate good control. Resist the temptation to change any rules so that you can drink in different ways from those you initially specified. Doing this is a sign that moderate drinking may not be possible for you, and abstinence may be a better way to proceed.

Paul is a 32-year-old, single man who found himself drinking uncontrollably on most weekends when out with his high school friends. He was also drinking several times during the week, so much so that he typically felt horrible the next morning, although he never missed work. He wanted to see if he could control his drinking and made a rule to not drink with his buddies, which meant that if he went out with them, he would not drink. While it was suggested that it would be very difficult to see his friends and not drink, he simply could not fathom no longer socializing with them.

For two weeks, Paul saw his friends and didn't drink. However, in his third week of trying to control his drinking, they ended up at a bar, where he had several drinks. While he knew that this violated his moderate drinking contract, he felt good that he was able to limit himself to three drinks, and without informing me he changed his contract to allow himself to drink with these friends and to have at most three drinks. Two weeks later, though, he went out with his friends and his drinking again got totally out of control.

Paul had changed his contract to accommodate his drinking and wish to drink before he had successfully demonstrated that he could hold to his current drinking contract. Through this experience, Paul not only learned that he couldn't go out with his friends and drink, but also that he simply couldn't socialize with them when drinking was part of the picture. He changed his contract again, but this time it contained the rule to never socialize with his high school friends in group settings where alcohol was consumed.

When You Can Change Your Rules. You can modify your drinking rules *if you are able to easily and successfully hold to your controlled drinking contract for a period of at least three months.* Such a decision should be well thought out, and changes should not be made on the spur of the moment. And again, the new contract must clearly specify guidelines that will govern all aspects of your drinking, just like your initial contract did. In addition, you must continue to closely monitor your drinking to see if the change in your drinking rules affects your ability to successfully control your drinking. If it does, you obviously need to tighten the rules again and to provide more structure for yourself.

Jim, a 40-year-old former client of mine, became worried because he had noticed a pattern of increased drinking over the course of the past year, to the point that he was drinking almost every day after work and hiding it from his family. In fact, his wife, Ellen, was surprised when he told her that he thought he had a drinking problem and that he had made the decision to stop drinking. Prior to his escalated pattern of drinking, he enjoyed drinking, but only on weekends and very occasionally during the week. He made the decision to stop drinking and was able to achieve abstinence fairly easily.

After about three months, he began to miss drinking, and he wished that he could occasionally have a glass of wine or a beer with his wife when they went out to dinner on weekends. He decided that he would attempt to moderate his drinking rather than to completely abstain, and he made a drinking contract that permitted him to drink only on Friday and Saturday nights when he was with his wife. In addition, when he drank, he would have at most two glasses of wine or two beers.

He was able to do this without difficulty, and after another three months, he wondered if he could also drink with some of his and his wife's friends. There were several couples with whom they tended to socialize, and the couples had always drunk socially together. Until now, Jim and his wife had continued to see these other couples, but he did not drink. As he had been very successful with his current moderate drinking contract, and it did not appear to be a struggle for him to hold to it, he modified his contract. His new contract allowed him still to drink only on weekends, but he also permitted himself to drink when he socialized with their mutual friends. He also increased his consumption from at most two to three drinks. This change did not lead to any difficulties for Jim, and he continued to successfully control his drinking.

Elizabeth was a 30-year-old woman who had been married to Gary for four years and had a two-year-old daughter. She came to see me because she was getting more and more concerned about her drinking, which she did almost every day to relax. But what worried her most was her heavier drinking, which took place on the weekends with a group of her and her husband's friends. She would get quite intoxicated and started experiencing blackouts. There were even times when she embarrassed herself due to her drunkenness. The next day, her friends often told her how drunk she had been, mentioning that there were times when she had barely made sense when she had spoken. While she knew she had been inebriated, she had no idea how drunk she truly had been. Even though her husband wasn't particularly concerned about her drinking, it still bothered Elizabeth. The couple worked full time, and Elizabeth was the primary caretaker of her daughter in the evenings, when Gary attended school.

Elizabeth's parents were heavy drinkers, and she wondered

whether she was an alcoholic. But over the past three weeks she had only drunk on a couple of occasions and only had two beers each time, so she wondered if she could moderate her drinking.

In our session, Elizabeth decided to drink at most three times per week, and at most three beers when she drank. She limited herself to beer because, when she lost control of her drinking, she drank mixed vodka drinks. She didn't think that there were any situations that she needed to avoid completely to not lose control of her drinking, and she thought if she stuck to beer, she could still socialize with her and her husband's friends in heavy drinking social situations. She also decided to start exercising in the evenings as a way to relax.

During the next week, Elizabeth not only held to her contract, but she didn't even have all three drinks, sometimes having only two. For three months, things remain unchanged, and Elizabeth wondered if she could drink on four days if she continued to limit the number of her drinks each week to nine (and no more than three on one day), which was the total weekly amount in her original contract. She also would never drink more than three drinks at any one time. She revised her contract, and for seven months she held to it without problems. There were even many weeks when she didn't drink on all four days, and she continued her pattern of exercising in the evenings. She was actually amused by how she used to get so intoxicated, and she enjoyed her new identity as a moderate drinker. Getting so drunk simply became unacceptable to her.

3. The Contract Is Forever

A contract that specifies safe drinking for you is essential to maintain. Your drinking has been a problem, and vigilance is needed to ensure that you continue to moderate your drinking and that it doesn't again become excessive. Your moderate drinking contract is a reminder that you need to be mindful of how you drink and that you are not a social drinker. The possibility of again experiencing alcohol-related problems is real, and you must be on guard.

I have seen people moderate their drinking for years with little difficulty and increase their upper limit to four drinks without experiencing a loss of control or any alcohol-related problems. These people still, though, did not drink more than one drink per hour, and they continued to remain mindful of the possibility of drinking too much. In addition, they typically did not drink all four drinks.

I also have observed people who, after the same amount of time of successfully moderating their drinking, *occasionally* allowed themselves to drink a little more, sometimes five or six drinks, such as when they attended a get-together that lasted many hours, from the afternoon into the evening. These were, though, very occasional and special events, and at other times these people were in control enough to continue to hold to their usual limits. They also maintained other features of their moderate drinking contract, such as never drinking more than three or four times per week and remembering to pace themselves when they drank.

For these individuals, drinking in controlled ways through adherence to their contract became more or less their norm, and over time, they were able to moderate their drinking with less effort. It became their way of life.

WRITING YOUR MODERATE DRINKING CONTRACT

Now you have a good sense of how to moderate your drinking. The next step is to complete your moderate drinking contract, which can be found at the end of this chapter. Since your moderate drinking contract needs to be based upon your unique drinking pattern, here's what to do:

Get a pen, turn to the contract at the end of this chapter (or make a copy of it), and begin. Be cautious and conservative. Your drinking has been out of control, and your chances of success will be improved if you are careful and vigilant.

1. Circle the maximum number of drinks that you will ever drink in one sitting.
2. Write down the type of alcohol you will drink.
3. Circle the maximum number of times during one week you will drink.

Next, think carefully about your pattern of drinking.

4. Write down examples of the specific situations in which you have been able to control your drinking. These will be the only situations in which you can drink (your low-risk situations).
5. Write down the situations—settings, places, bars, times—in which you have lost control of your drinking. In these situations, you will never drink again (your high-risk situations).
6. Write down the social settings you need to completely avoid, because despite your best intentions, you will not be able to resist drinking and drinking too much in those situations.

After you are satisfied with your moderate drinking contract, show it to the people who are most concerned about you and your drinking to help gain their support.

Now is the time to place all of your energy into moderating your drinking. You've thought long and hard about your pattern of alcohol use, and you've developed a personal moderate drinking contract that outlines rules to govern your drinking. It's now up to you to follow your contract religiously so that you can start to feel better about yourself and avoid any alcohol-related problems. I recommend reviewing chapter 7, as the general techniques I outlined in that chapter are critically important to follow.

Over time, if you have been able to control your drinking without much difficulty, you may modify your moderate drinking contract, but this should only occur if you have been able to hold to it without difficulty for a period of three months. Again, the new contract needs to specify rules concerning your drinking just as the old one did. At all times, your drinking must fall within the limits that you have specified. If it does not, you are not moderating your drinking, and you need to go back to the original moderate drinking contract that had been working for you.

MY MODERATE DRINKING CONTRACT

1. When I drink, I *at most* will drink:

      one drink   two drinks   three drinks   four drinks.

2. I will *only* drink the following types of alcohol: _____

3. During a week, I *at most* will drink: once   twice   three times   four times

4. I will *only* drink in the following situations (be as specific as possible):

_____

_____

_____

_____

_____

_____

5. I will *never* drink in the following situations (be as specific as possible):

_____

_____

_____

6. Situations I will completely avoid are (be as specific as possible):

_____

_____

_____

**** If I cannot successfully control my drinking, I will make the decision to stop drinking entirely.

_____

                      Signature

9

BUMPS AND DETOURS WITH MODERATE DRINKING

The road to success is always under construction.

ARNOLD PALMER

When you try to moderate your drinking, some bumps will inevitably arise. You may find yourself sometimes drinking more than what you agreed to in your moderate drinking contract, or you may sometimes drink more often than what you wrote in your contract. If you violate *any* rule regarding the amount or frequency of drinking specified in your moderate drinking contract, this violation is a cause for concern that needs to be addressed. While this doesn't necessarily signal that you are not able to drink moderately, it does mean that you should take a closer look at why you felt the need to drink more and consider whether abstinence should be your next step. And, regardless of how often or how much you drink, if your drinking causes you serious problems, such as finding yourself drinking and driving or getting into fights, abstinence must be considered as well.

KNOWING WHETHER YOUR CONTRACT
IS WORKING

Some problems that commonly occur when trying to moderate drinking follow, along with suggestions regarding how to address them. If you see yourself in any of these scenarios, and if problems continue even with some adjustments in your moderate drinking contract, you should seriously consider abstinence.

Can You Succeed in Your Contract at All?

The best indicator of whether moderate drinking is working for you is whether or not you remain in control. It's not uncommon for some problems to occur during this learning process. The trick is to learn from setbacks so you can avoid them in the future as you continue on the path to resolving your drinking problem.

That said, you need to understand that your goal should be to succeed, especially during the first couple of months. It's not a positive sign if you have only limited success during this time, and setbacks mean that abstinence is probably a better way for you to go.

Kevin, a married 32-year-old man, was a heavy drinker who drank almost every day. During the week, he would drink about a six-pack each night, and on the weekends, he could easily drink 10 to 15 beers in a day. He came to see me due to pressure from his wife, Debby, who was very concerned about his drinking. Kevin wanted to try to moderate his drinking, so he decided that he would drink a maximum of four beers at any one sitting and would only drink three times a week. I met with Kevin and Debby, and while Debby expressed her concern about Kevin's ability to drink moderately, she was willing to support his plan. Kevin's drinking generally took place at home, but on the weekends he and Debby often went out to clubs, either alone or with friends. We discussed changing their pattern of going to clubs on the weekends, since that is where Kevin's heaviest drinking took place, but Kevin believed he could control his drinking in those settings.

When I saw Kevin one week later and he reported that although he was able to drink less than he had been, he could not hold to his contract. Kevin drank four times that week and over-drank on two of the occasions, having 8 and 10 beers. As he was out at a bar when he over-drank, I suggested that Kevin either not drink at all or avoid going to bars. Kevin didn't want to hear this and stated that he simply needed to try harder.

The next week, he reported more lapses in his contract. He had drunk on five days, not his agreed-upon four. On one of those days he had only had two beers, but on two days he drank seven beers at a bar. It was only then that Kevin decided that it was best not to drink at all when he went out. Unfortunately, he was unable to adhere to this decision. Over the next several weeks he decided to stop going to clubs and bars altogether, but he couldn't hold to this either. Only then could Kevin come to the conclusion that moderating his drinking just wasn't possible, and we worked out a plan of abstinence. If you, like Kevin, have only limited success in holding to your moderate drinking contract, particularly when you first try to do it, take it as a sign that moderate drinking is not possible for you.

How Far Over Your Limit Did You Go?

If you violated your contract, did drinking get totally out of hand or was it more modest? Did controlled drinking escalate to uncontrolled drinking? By this I mean, did you find yourself downing five drinks when your rule was to drink no more than three? Or did you polish off eight, 10, or 15 drinks instead of the three? Obviously, if you are that out of control, moderate drinking is not working for you. The same can be said if you are drinking and driving or if your use of alcohol caused you another kind of serious problem.

But if your drinking was not completely out of control, but still nonetheless exceeded your self-imposed limit, it might make sense, at least for now, for you to continue to try moderating your drinking.

THREE WAYS TO MAKE STICKING TO YOUR LIMITS EASIER

1. Change Your Social Scene

Drinking and heavy drinking are partly influenced by your social setting. When you first developed your moderate drinking contract, you needed to determine the types of situations that trigger you to drink excessively. These were the situations you decided to not drink in or to avoid completely.

It is also possible that you made a mistake when you first developed your moderate drinking contract because you overlooked what was for you a high-risk setting. If you have exceeded your drinking limit and you feel the setting might have played a role in this, consider it off-limits and think about whether it would be best for you to avoid drinking in it or to avoid it completely.

Karen, a 44-year-old successful businesswoman, first began drinking in high school. According to Karen, in high school and throughout her 20s she only drank lightly on Friday and Saturday nights. In her 30s, perhaps influenced by the friends she socialized with, she began drinking more heavily and on the weekends often found herself driving home at night after having had too much to drink. In fact, one evening she was pulled over by the police after drinking, but fortunately (or unfortunately), she did not get arrested for drunk driving because she was not tested. Karen's drinking now extended to the weekdays as well. This was compounded by her job, which required a fair amount of business travel and socializing with business associates. The amount of alcohol she was consuming started to concern her, and she worried about how her drinking could be affecting her health.

Karen's drinking contract specified that she would only drink on Friday and Saturday nights and *at most* once during the week, with a maximum limit of three drinks a night. I expressed concern about whether she could control her weekend drinking when she went out with her friends. Karen felt that she could, and she even decided to talk with her friends about her plan to limit her drinking. Over the next few weeks, Karen proved me wrong and easily held to her moderate drinking contract. Feeling great about her progress, we decided that she didn't need to see me for two months, and then just to see how things were going.

At that meeting, Karen reported that to her surprise there had been several times when she drank too much. While she had only rarely exceeded the number of times each week she was allowed to drink, it was the amount she drank that really concerned her. Karen's drinking had on several occasions reached six drinks. As we analyzed this pattern more closely, it was obvious that each time she had violated her moderate drinking contract, she had been away on a business trip. In the evenings, she met her business associates in the hotel lounge, and it was during these times that she either drank too much or drank when she had planned not to drink.

When Karen first developed her moderate drinking contract, she didn't even consider the evenings of her business trips. She believed that she would meet her colleagues in the hotel lounge and would simply not drink or would drink on just one of the evenings. She also believed that she could limit her drinking in this situation, which proved more difficult than she initially thought. Karen revised her moderate drinking contract to specify that while on a business trip, she would go to the lounge only once during the entire trip. On the nights she didn't go to the lounge, she worked out in the fitness club or stayed in her room and watched a movie or read a book. In addition, when she did go out on that one night, she would arrive later and would have, at most, one drink. This worked for Karen, and she was able to achieve success with her new moderate drinking contract.

Then there was Rob, single and 28 years old, who found that he would drink too much during his weekly poker game with friends. Instead of holding to his four-drink limit, he would commonly have five or six. Rob knew his poker game might be a problem when he first developed his moderate drinking contract, yet he allowed himself this social activity. Despite his repeated attempts to control his drinking by leaving early (which he never managed to do), or by waiting to have his first drink (which he occasionally did), he was not successful and eventually made the decision to drop his poker game. He found it impossible to go there and not over-drink, so he needed to modify his moderate drinking contract to make this setting off-limits.

Both Rob and Karen were able not only to look at their drinking patterns but also to change. The key here is to be honest with yourself and to remain focused on adhering to your contract, which must be placed ahead of your desire to have a drink.

There are also people who despite listing certain situations as high-risk settings to completely avoid, have found themselves in those social settings and lost control of their drinking. They eventually learned that they could not consistently avoid those situations (and keep their drinking in control), so they chose abstinence. If you find that this occurs with you, you'll need to give up on the idea of moderating your drinking.

2. Be Careful What You Drink

What type of alcoholic beverage were you drinking when things turned excessive? As stated in the last chapter, some people find that they cannot control their drinking with a certain type of alcohol. If in your initial moderate drinking contract you did not specify the type of permitted alcohol, but you later discover that a certain type of alcohol is problematic for you, it makes sense to modify your contract to change to a beverage that you may not have a problem with. Jason, for example, discovered that he could control his drinking by drinking only beer and never drinking hard liquor at all, even in mixed drinks.

For others, the type of alcohol is irrelevant because regardless of what they drink, they cannot control their alcohol use. If this describes you, abstinence is your only route to recovery.

3. Limit How Much You Drink

In your original moderate drinking contract, you needed to specify the maximum number of drinks you would have whenever you drank. You may have decided on four, but in reality, that amount may be too much for you. It is easy for that many drinks to turn into five or even six. Consider limiting even further how much you drink at any one time. Try to drink at most three, or even two, to see if that helps you to stick to your limits. With that added structure, moderation will be easier.

If you drink at home, limit the amount of alcohol you have. For example, if you decided to drink at most three beers, only have three beers at home and don't have the whole six-pack or case. Again, that structure may help you to moderate how much you drink. If these things, don't help, the answer for you is abstinence.

DO YOU DRINK MORE OFTEN THAN THE RULE IN YOUR CONTRACT?

Even if your drinking does not get totally out of control, rules can still be violated. A rule violation means drinking more often than you specified in your contract. For instance, instead of drinking three times per week, you drink four, five, or six times.

Think about your inability to comply with your moderate drinking contract. Do you often drink more frequently than your rule specifies, or is this an occasional occurrence? An occasional violation means that your drinking exceeds the rule a few times a year. A frequent violation is anything more, whether it be monthly, weekly, or even more often. Quite simply, you cannot exceed the limits you have set for yourself. A slip-up once, twice, or even three times a year is acceptable—you are human—provided your drinking did not cause you serious difficulties. Any more than that and you should consider abstinence.

TWO WAYS TO AVOID DRINKING TOO OFTEN

1. Think about and Change Your Surroundings

Just as the context and social setting in which you drink is very important in limiting the amount of alcohol you drink at a time, the same principles apply to the number of times you drink each week. Even if your drinking does not exceed your limit in terms of the amount, if you find yourself drinking more often than you originally specified, you may need to examine when you increased your frequency.

Bob, 26 years old and single, decided that he was only going to drink three times each week, but he found that he regularly drank five or six times. When he looked closely at this pattern, he discovered that whenever he got together with a certain group of friends after work, he tended to drink. He was also in a bowling league where the members consistently drank, and this also made it easy for him to go beyond his three times per week limit. He eventually made the decision to quit his bowling league and to see his drinking buddies less often. While Bob's friends were important to him, as was his bowling, his drinking problem was an even more important priority.

Brenda, a single mom, found that her drinking increased from three times a week to four or five times if alcohol was available at her house. Her leisure time involved simply winding down at home after work, and while she couldn't change that, she could change having alcohol so readily available to her in this situation. She decided to have limited amounts of alcohol in the home only on the days when she allowed herself to drink, and this structure helped her to stick to her three-day-per-week rule.

If your own drinking exceeds your rules in terms of how often you drink, try to figure out why this is happening. There are, no doubt, situations you need to avoid that you hadn't thought about before you made your contract, and now is the time to make these changes. If you still continue to drink too often no matter how you to try to modify your contract, abstinence will be your best and only choice. It is just that simple.

2. Limit How Often You Drink

You may also need to re-evaluate the number of times each week you allow yourself to drink. The maximum number of days anyone should drink in a week is four, and drinking on four days may not provide you with enough structure. Four days easily can expand to five or six. If you decided to drink on four days but you're having trouble holding to this limit, try decreasing your maximum number of days to two or three. The increased structure may help you to better moderate your drinking.

Mark originally decided that he would drink on Friday and Saturday nights and twice during the week. However, before long, he found himself drinking Thursday through Sunday, and then occasionally on other weekdays as well. For him, changing the number of times he could drink to only two gave him the increased structure he needed.

LIMITING ALCOHOL ISN'T ALWAYS EASY

If you have successfully moderated your intake, how difficult is it to do? Do you still enjoy drinking, or is the hassle of limiting your intake making drinking no longer pleasurable? Is it a struggle to avoid everyday drinking or to reduce your drinking to only three or four times each week? Do you find yourself wanting to drink more than you are allowed? Are you wondering if it is worth the effort and struggle?

For some people, moderating drinking is not a constant effort, and for some, it may even be fairly easy. However, if this is not the case for you and moderating alcohol intake becomes an unpleasant experience, it makes sense for you to try abstinence. Why? Because moderating your drinking should not be unpleasant. The benefits to your life as a result of drinking less should start to outweigh and outnumber the problems that drinking causes for you. Think long and hard about this. Remember, your only choices are moderation or abstinence. Drinking more is not an option.

MODERATION DOESN'T ALWAYS WORK, AND THAT'S OKAY

One of the most common scenarios among problem drinkers is difficulty acknowledging that they cannot moderate their drinking. You may try and try to limit your alcohol consumption, but with only very limited success. You may wish to be like those who can drink without problems, but this is simply that: *a wish.*

It's when you believe that statement that you're on the road to getting better. Moderate drinking may not have succeeded the way you first thought and hoped it would. But it has succeeded nonetheless, because it proved to you that your use of alcohol cannot be moderated and that abstinence needs to be the way for you to resolve your alcohol problem.

IT COMES DOWN TO MODERATION OR ABSTINENCE

The decision to give up on moderate drinking and instead pursue a course of abstinence is a tough one. *But this is what you need to do if you want alcohol to stop interfering with your life.* The evidence is clear: If alcohol continues to hurt you, even though you are trying your best to moderate your drinking, you need to give it up entirely.

Some people just cannot moderate their drinking, despite their best efforts. Don't be down on yourself. Accept this fact, and I promise you that it won't be long before you see how true this advice is. Make the decision to stop drinking completely and see how your life improves.

Sean is a 32-year-old married man, father of one-year-old twins. Sean had been a "heavy partier" during high school and in his 20s. Sean could easily drink 15 beers during the course of an evening, and sometimes even more. He and his friends were all into the heavy drinking scene, and on many nights they tended to congregate at one of several local bars, drinking quite heavily and staying until very late. Prior to getting married, Sean wasn't particularly concerned about his drinking, as he had few other responsibilities and partying was an integral part of his life.

Now, five years after his marriage, Sean had slowed down his drinking, but he still drank quite heavily at the bars on many nights, sometimes with his wife, Ann, who is a light drinker, and at other times without her. After Ann gave birth to their twins, Sean's heavy drinking began to become more of an issue. While Ann stayed home caring for their children, Sean was out drinking. There were times on the weekends when Sean got so drunk that the next day he was totally useless to help Ann out with child care. When his drinking started to affect his relationship with Ann, Sean got concerned.

Sean drew the line at abstinence and preferred to try to moderate his drinking. He decided that he would drink at most four beers per occasion and would only drink on Friday and Saturday nights and once during the week. He still wanted to be able to drink with his friends at the local bars, and he thought that he could control his drinking there.

The next week, Sean reported that his success had been mixed.

While he only drank three times, on one evening at the bar, he drank way too much and got home very late, which caused an argument with Ann. However, on the other weekend night when he was out with Ann at the bar, he was able to limit his drinking. He then revised his contract to allow himself to drink at bars only when he was with Ann. He would still go to bars by himself, but on those times, he would not drink alcohol.

This revision, unfortunately, didn't work for long. Sean started drinking in bars without Ann and ended up getting drunk and getting home very late. He then decided that he would never go to a bar without Ann, and he revised his contract to reflect this. That, too, did not work, because after going out with Ann, drinking a little too much, and returning home with her, he would go back out and get very drunk.

Even after all this, Sean still would not consider abstinence. As a last-ditch effort at moderation, he decided that the *only* time he would ever drink was when he went out to dinner with Ann. There, they often would split a bottle of wine, and that never seemed to present a problem for him. He also decided that he would never go to another bar, as he simply could not control his drinking in that setting. We discussed the idea of his doing some limited drinking while home, but Sean never drank at home and had no desire to start. So his contract was now modified so that he was only able to drink on the weekends when out to dinner with Ann (where they would split one bottle of wine) and he would never go to a bar alone or with friends.

Despite his contract, over the next couple of months, Sean reverted to occasionally going to bars and getting very intoxicated. I'm happy to say that Sean finally admitted that the only way he was going to solve his drinking problem was abstinence. After he made this decision, his life began to improve.

HOW BUMPS AND DETOURS CAN WORK TO YOUR ADVANTAGE

The process of trying to moderate your drinking may be something you needed to do. Discovering that you can't drink moderately is actually a positive development. You learned a lot about yourself and your relationship to alcohol, and you now know that you need to stop drinking completely to resolve your drinking problem. If you didn't go through this process, you would always wonder if you could moderate your drinking, and this would make it difficult for you to commit to abstinence to resolve your drinking problem. So your journey has given you knowledge and information and has solidified in your mind what you now must do—achieve abstinence from alcohol.

THE TRANSITION TO QUITTING

While moderating drinking represents a lifestyle change, quitting drinking is an even bigger one. But try not to feel overwhelmed. Many, many people learn to quit drinking and still love life. In fact, many learned to love life even more without drinking—and so will you. I have even heard some say that learning to live life without alcohol was the best thing that ever happened to them. So don't be scared by what you are facing. Instead, view it as a new journey and an opportunity for growth.

☐ ☐ ☐

You know now whether or not moderation is working for you. If you encountered some bumps along the way, but have learned from these experiences and modified your drinking contract to enable you to achieve success, great! In fact, some bumps are inevitable and give you insight into your pattern of drinking and what traps you need to be on guard for. The key is learning from these experiences so you don't step into the same traps over and over.

However, if you keep experiencing bumps and your drinking problems continue no matter how you modify your contract, you have learned that abstinence needs to be your next step. And that's okay. The next four chapters will help you to stop drinking entirely.

Facts do not cease to exist because they are ignored.
ALDOUS HUXLEY

PART IV

QUITTING DRINKING AND STAYING SOBER

10

MANAGING YOUR THOUGHTS
TO QUIT DRINKING

*Self-disciplined begins with the mastery of your
thoughts. If you don't control what you think, you
can't control what you do. Simply, self-discipline
enables you to think first and act afterward.*

NAPOLEON HILL

I'm sure that your decision to stop drinking has not been easy. Drinking has been an important part of your life, and the idea of quitting may be a little scary. But now you realize that you cannot moderate your drinking and that abstinence is the only way to stop alcohol from ruining your life. You may even have tried to moderate your drinking by reading this book and were not successful. Regardless of how you have reached the decision to abstain from alcohol, you must now learn to avoid drinking and commit to yourself to making this a reality.

There are many proven techniques that will help you not pick up that first drink and that will make quitting alcohol much less stressful. These techniques can be learned in the privacy of your home rather than by going to AA or other self-help meetings, psychiatrists, psychologists, alcohol counselors, or more intensive treatment programs. Whether you consider your drinking problem a disease or a bad habit does not matter, as these techniques will help you regardless of how you understand why you can't control your drinking. The only thing that matters is your commitment and desire to stop drinking.

The fact that you know you need to completely abstain from alcohol to resolve your drinking problem suggests that your problem with alcohol is somewhat serious. As I mentioned in chapter 5, alcohol problems can damage your body, and I would strongly encourage you to see your doctor to get checked out. In the event that you have any medical conditions that have been caused or worsened by your drinking, you should know this so that you can get them treated. In addition, some people with more severe alcohol problems have emotional problems as well, whether these are feelings of anxiety, extreme moodiness, or just feeling down in the dumps. If these problems are not treated, they can make the process of getting sober more difficult. So, if you experience these kinds of feelings, talk with your doctor about them. He or she can refer you for psychological counseling, which I review in chapter 16, or to a psychiatrist who can evaluate the need for psychiatric medication, which I review in more detail in chapter 17. While you may not need medication, it is a good idea to at least get this checked out so that you know for certain. With that being said, let's now review ways for you to think about your alcohol problem that will help you and make the whole process of quitting alcohol easier.

YOU ARE NOT ALONE!

The idea of no longer drinking is probably very unsettling to you. It signals a major change in the way you live your life, and you may even believe that you are in an extreme minority. The idea that most everyone drinks, except you and others who have made the decision to stop, can make you feel isolated, alone, and different. But you shouldn't think that you are missing out on something by abstaining. If drinking was so great, why did it cause you so much grief? You're quitting so that you *won't* miss out on anything in life.

If you're falling into the familiar trap of thinking that most everyone drinks but you, it's because alcohol has been central to most of your social activities for much of your life. You may be very surprised to learn that many, many people do not drink at all. Research in the United States has shown that about 48 percent of adults completely abstain from alcohol or drink fewer than 12 drinks per year. As you enter a non-drinking lifestyle, you'll experience this first hand. These non-drinkers live fulfilled and happy lives. Not drinking is simply a lifestyle choice; it does not need to be as big of an issue as you may think. Sure, you need to adjust to this, as it represents a big change for you, but it is a choice you won't regret making. So let's get on with it. Stopping drinking is not easy, but drinking the way you have hasn't been easy either. Remember that you aren't alone. Like others, you will learn to enjoy life without drinking.

NOT TO DRINK: YOUR NUMBER 1 PRIORITY

Make Not Drinking Your Daily Thought

Every day, consciously take the time to remember that you are trying to change your life by not taking even one drink.

When you wake up every morning, remind yourself by saying out loud, "*Today* I am choosing not to drink." This is your first step to sobriety. You'll succeed if you remember to keep your not-drinking decision in the forefront of your mind. You must live and breathe this thought, all day and every day. Abstinence is your goal for today. Then, plan your day with activities that do not include drinking. Here's how.

Planning a Life without Alcohol

When you first stop drinking, plan your day around avoiding all alcohol-related activities. Be prepared, anticipate, carefully evaluate, and avoid any situation that can potentially endanger your abstinence.

For example, if your friends suggest stopping off for a drink after work, don't try to convince yourself that you can go with them and not drink. Instead, find a pleasant way to decline the invitation. If you are invited to play cards or for a barbecue, and you believe that drinking will be a part of the social setting, you should also decline because of the possibility that you might be tempted to drink.

Making the decision to avoid former problem situations is not easy, and you will not be able to foresee every temptation. If your goal of not drinking, however, is your number 1 thought, you will be prepared to make these decisions.

As you become more comfortable in your new role as a non-drinker, you'll be able to participate in more activities where alcohol is served. But for now, it's best to avoid these activities altogether.

Be Prepared with Excuses

You may want to think in advance about what to say when you decline an invitation. At times you may feel comfortable saying that you are trying to stop drinking and that you're turning down their offer because you would be too tempted to drink. In other situations you may feel more comfortable offering an excuse of having other plans or other things to do. Feel free to say different things to different people depending upon how well you know them or the type of relationship you have with them. There is no right or wrong way to decline; just say what feels right for you at the time. Your explanations may change as you gain comfort in your decision not to drink.

Focus on the Benefits of Not Drinking

It is important to try not to dwell on what you are not doing or what you think you are missing. Instead, focus on the positive benefits of no longer drinking and how your life is improving (no fights with your spouse, you're alert and prepared at the office, you're saving money by not buying alcohol, you feel better physically, you have less guilt, you're no longer drinking and driving, etc.).

In chapter 3, you thought about and wrote down all of the benefits that you will obtain by changing your relationship to alcohol. Now is the time to focus on and remain mindful of these. Remembering these benefits will help to keep you concentrated on why you have made the decision to stop drinking.

ONE DAY AT A TIME

Alcoholics Anonymous encourages taking things "one day at a time," and this is a good strategy for you, too. Here's how it works: think about not drinking for *today* and for *today only*. This strategy is much more manageable than thinking about not drinking for the rest of your life, which may be too overwhelming for you right now. Instead, try to live with the thought, "I am not drinking today," and then do everything in your power not to drink between morning and bedtime. You can even break it down into smaller chunks of time if you need to. For example, if your pattern was to go for a drink after work, you can tell yourself, "tonight, for the next five hours, I am not going to drink."

One-day-at-a-time thinking also can be useful when you encounter other difficult situations in your life, including financial hardship, a relationship breakup, a medical problem, or other troubles. Particularly when you first abstain from alcohol, problems may feel overwhelming and impossible to bear without a drink. This is because you probably have not developed all of the coping skills you need, since you used to use alcohol as a way to cope. During these times, it can be helpful to remember that all you really need to do is get through the day.

Less Is More, So Small Steps Lead to Big Changes

Again, you can break your periods of abstinence into even smaller units, such as one hour at a time or even minutes at a time. If you segment your time this way, it will be much easier for you to deal with almost any temptation to take a drink. Here's why: The shorter the time, the easier it is to avoid temptation from almost any compulsive activity, whether it is smoking, eating unhealthy food, or drinking alcohol. Keeping this up for the rest of your life may seem overwhelming and impossible, but the next hour or the next half hour is easily doable and sometimes long enough for the urge to drink to pass. And that's the whole point, one small hurdle at a time.

Bob found that "keeping it in the day" was the main thing he needed to do to remain abstinent. "All I need to remember is to not drink today . . . and only today. Tomorrow isn't anything I need to worry or think about. Tomorrow turns into today and I only think about that when it comes and never before."

You may question this "one-day-at-a-time" philosophy and think that it is childlike and that long-range planning is important. It is true that many goals are best achieved by taking into account the long-range, global picture (saving money, buying a home, and setting up a business are some examples). However, when it comes to stopping or changing a compulsive activity like drinking, the one-day-at-a-time philosophy really works.

For example, let's assume that it is August, and you have decided to stop drinking. Don't think now about not being able to drink when you celebrate Thanksgiving or New Year's Eve, or your friend's bachelor party next year. That kind of thinking will overwhelm you and bring you down. Instead, deal with today and cope with these future events as they happen. You will probably find that when those events come around, not drinking will be no big deal.

Stay in the Present

Remember that you will think and feel differently in the future than you do now. While the idea of not being able to drink on New Year's Eve might sound dreadful in August, when New Year's Eve comes, and you have some abstinence under your belt and you have learned to enjoy your life without needing a drink, not drinking may not even be an issue. Worry about and think about tomorrow only when tomorrow comes . . . and never before.

Scott stopped drinking in September and was very worried about celebrating Christmas with his family. Getting together for Christmas was the family ritual, and everyone drank heavily at that time. In October, Scott just didn't know how he was going to handle this. Should he go? Not go? If he didn't go, how would his family feel? Could he go and not drink? He even wondered if he could enjoy Christmas at all without drinking. Scott finally decided that he would worry about this in two months when Christmas came, and in the meantime he simply focused on not drinking in the present. And when Christmas arrived, he found that how to celebrate wasn't even a big issue! He decided to stop by his family's home for a fairly brief period of time, and he spent most of the evening with his wife, Sarah, starting a new tradition—driving around looking at the Christmas lights and then having a quiet, romantic evening at home.

Feeling Better Happens One Day at a Time

Remember that once you stop drinking, it will take time before you begin to feel better. So don't be discouraged if your life doesn't turn around immediately as soon as you stop drinking.

Even though your drinking has stopped, the damage that alcohol has done to you may be present for a long time. Your relationships may still be filled with tension and conflict. You may continue to experience job-related difficulties, or you may be dealing with drink-related legal problems. Or perhaps you are seeing your life with a clear head for the first time in a long time, and you do not like what you see. It is now that you must be strong, because any of these kinds of scenarios can lead you back to drinking. But don't retreat. Drinking may seem like the easier option, but it's not. If you drink, in time, problems will only compound, your health will suffer, and your relationships will deteriorate. Staying abstinent is the best choice. Harder now, maybe, but well worth it for a happy, healthy future.

Recovering from a drinking problem occurs one day at a time. It can and will take time to get your life back to where you would like it to be. If you have been drinking for 20 years, it may take more than a few weeks, or even a few months, to begin to feel really good about your life, but things will get a bit better every day.

Try to not get frustrated. You have made the commitment not to drink. Success will be within your grasp if you keep that priority clearly in your mind and remember that you *will* begin to feel better, but only one day at a time.

Time Is a Healer

It may sound like a cliché, but time is an amazing healer. What seems unbearable now will not be in the future. In time, you will develop additional coping skills and a greater ability to deal with whatever happens. Meeting difficulties one day at a time and just getting through the day can often be enormously useful. Deal with your future when it comes and not before.

NEVER FORGET THE CONSEQUENCES OF YOUR DRINKING

Although some parts of drinking were enjoyable, other parts had a destructive impact on your life. *Wanting to avoid the consequences of drinking is the primary reason you decided to do something about your drinking problem.* Always remain mindful of the pain your drinking has caused and will continue to cause you if you return to it.

It is very common for ex-drinkers to minimize the extent of their past drinking. They begin to think that their problem wasn't so bad. When they crave a drink, they may actually forget about their past difficulties. The mind has an amazing ability to forget pain and to play tricks on us. Don't let this happen to you.

Write a List of Harmful Consequences and Review It Daily

Write a list of the harm drinking has caused you and others. Spend time thinking of all of the ways drinking has hurt you, affected your sense of self and self-esteem, or hurt your relationships with others. Keep this list handy for quick reference and review it daily to keep the pain fresh in your mind. You should also often reread the cons of your drinking in the *Pros and Cons of Drinking* exercise that you completed in chapter 3. Doing this will keep you focused on the reasons why you have decided to stop drinking.

This exercise is not meant to make you feel bad; rather, it is intended to help you to remember why you made the commitment to no longer drink. The harm and bad feelings caused by past drinking must remain alive in your mind. If you begin to forget why you stopped drinking, this list can be a very useful reminder to you. Particularly when you first stop drinking, make it a *daily habit* to review this to help you to remain focused on why you are no longer drinking and to remember what will occur if you start drinking again.

ABSTINENCE IS ABSTINENCE — FOREVER

You already know that you can't moderate your drinking and that abstinence is the only way to recover from your drinking problem. You've probably tried dozens of times, if not more, to control your drinking, and because you couldn't do this, you're now committed to staying sober. So why am I telling you that abstinence is abstinence— forever? You know this, right? Here's why:

After a period of successful abstinence, it is *extremely* common to begin to think that you can drink again, because you believe that it will be different this time around. You can admit that you drank too much in the past and lost control of your drinking, but this time you believe that you will be able to control your drinking and you won't allow it to take over your life. You tell yourself that with all you have learned, you will be able to drink safely and will *never* allow yourself to drink so much. This time, you will be careful and control your drinking. Wrong!

What Is One *Drink?*

Maybe you tell yourself that you will have *just one drink*. While you know that this holds the potential for difficulties, you believe that having just one drink won't hurt and will not escalate into more drinking. At the moment, you want to have a drink, and at the moment, you believe that it will cause no harm. After all, what's one drink?

Even One Drink Is Too Much

You've already proved to yourself that you cannot moderate your alcohol consumption, so one drink is never an option for you. In fact, for you, *any drinking will definitely lead to too much drinking.* Losing your commitment to not drink, and "forgetting" that you cannot drink any alcohol safely, will inevitably lead you back to abusive drinking. Beware. Once the door to your old behavior is slightly opened, it will eventually open all the way, and your drinking will again become excessive. Whatever your good intentions, you need to remember that this time will not be different. You are not able to moderate your drinking, and one drink is too much.

THERE'S NEVER A GOOD REASON TO DRINK

One of the easiest things to find is a reason to drink. Drinking can be justified for almost any reason:

- It was a good day.
- It was a bad day.

- It was a sunny day.
- It was a rainy day.
- You had a stressful day at work.
- You successfully closed on a deal you had been working on for months.
- Your favorite team won the Super Bowl.
- Your favorite team lost the Super Bowl.

It doesn't matter. If you want to drink, you can always find a reason. However, a *reason* to drink is simply an *excuse* to drink. In reality, there is never a reason to drink, and you need to be mindful that your brain will play tricks on you and try to convince you that there is.

Even Terrible Events Aren't Reasons to Drink

Life is filled with its ups and downs. On certain days, everything works out well, yet on other days, Murphy's Law applies. Nothing goes right, and you may begin to feel angry, frustrated, or resentful. When bad things happen and you feel angry, down, resentful, frustrated, or anxious, it's very tempting to tell yourself that you *deserve* a drink.

This is not in any way meant to minimize bad experiences such as a relationship breakup, getting diagnosed with a serious illness, or the death of someone close to you. Neither do I want to take lightly the feelings of intense anxiety or depression some people who are trying to stay sober experience and that may or may not even be related to events in their lives. However, no matter what happens or what you experience, *there is never a good reason for you to drink.* While you may believe that drinking can help you in the short term, it will only hurt you in the long term and eventually will make everything worse. Bob internalized a "zero-tolerance" policy. Regardless of what happened in his life, there was no place for drinking because he knew that "drinking would just mess everything up." Certainly, if you continue to be bothered by painful feelings, there are outside resources to help you, which I review in the final section of this book. Drinking, however, is not one of them.

⬜ ⬜ ⬜

You now know a lot of ways to think about your decision that will make it easier for you to not drink. In large part, your thoughts control your behavior, so you need to remember and incorporate these strategies into your daily thinking. It isn't easy to change our usual and automatic ways of thinking, so it is important that you practice the following:

- Remember that many people do not drink. You are not alone.
- Make no longer drinking your number 1 priority.
- Stop drinking one day at a time, or even an hour at a time, and worry about the future only when it comes.
- Focus on and never forget the consequences of your drinking.
- Keep in mind that one drink is too much, as it will open the door to out-of-control drinking. Abstinence is abstinence—forever.
- A reason to drink is only an excuse to drink. There is never a good reason to drink.

11

WHAT YOU MUST DO TO QUIT DRINKING

Activity is contagious.   RALPH WALDO EMERSON

In order to stop drinking, you will have to change not just the way you think, but also some of your behaviors. By this, I mean that your life needs to fill in the gap left by alcohol. You probably never realized how much of your day was either spent drinking or wasted because you were unable to function. The extra time you'll now have will be quite an adjustment, and you need to learn to fill it with things other than drinking, such as catching up with old friends, hanging out with your partner, playing with your kids, or finding a new hobby.

BOREDOM CAN LEAD BACK TO DRINKING

When you first stop drinking, it's common to feel like a fish out of water. You probably won't know what to do with yourself. This happens either because your drinking has replaced other previously familiar, pleasurable activities, or because with drinking the central focus of your life, you never even developed other leisure activities. Now you'll find that you can no longer participate in some activities that were a part of your drinking scenario (including, perhaps, spending time in bars, dart games, card games, bowling, watching a football game, and hanging out with particular friends), and this can lead to you feel bored. The danger is that your life can begin to seem dull and empty, which may lead you back to drinking. In fact, boredom is a big reason why people return to drinking after a period of abstinence. To stay the course and not drink, you must fill the void.

THE DRY DRUNK

Another danger is that even if you are able to stop drinking, but you don't fill the gap left by alcohol, you will feel miserable, bored, and empty, and you won't be happy about not drinking. And that's not good. The term "dry drunk" refers to the individual who is no longer drinking but who has not made any lifestyle changes. The dry drunk will feel resentful about not drinking and negative about life, and over time could even return to drinking. Dry drunks exhibit the same personality problems associated with active drinkers, except that now they aren't triggered by having a drink. Dry drunks are not fun to be around. You need to make real lifestyle changes in order to again love being alive and gain an optimistic outlook on life, laugh, love, plan for the future, and make time for friends and family. True recovery is the enjoyment of life without alcohol.

Think of your life as a pie. Alcohol, a big slice of that pie, has been cut out and removed. If you have the feeling that a big piece of your life is missing, you will feel pretty empty and bored. If you don't fill the void, you may remain abstinent, but you won't enjoy it. The key is discovering that your life is even more fulfilling and fun without drinking. It is critical that you keep busy, structure your day, and find fun things to do that don't include drinking, to avoid either returning to drinking or becoming a dry drunk.

STRUCTURE YOUR DAY AND MAKE PLANS

Every day, make a plan for the next day. Fill the times of the day when you used to drink with alcohol-free events. There are probably things you always wanted to do, places to see, or projects around the house that were not possible when drinking consumed your leisure time. Even something as enjoyable and simple as reading a book or going to a movie can stimulate you and take your mind off of alcohol. Plan ahead and hold to that plan. Faithfully staying with your schedule (as long as the scheduled plans do not include drinking) decreases your chances of returning to alcohol.

Filling in the Times When You Used to Drink

For example, let's assume you work from 9:00 am to 5:00 pm, and you commonly drank after work. The question is, what will you do from the time work lets out until bedtime? That's where planning ahead comes in. You should know what you are going to be doing that evening. Make it a point never to be in the situation of leaving work with no scheduled plans for the evening. These can be as simple as a trip to the supermarket, going to a bookstore, planning to watch a particular TV program, or cooking yourself (or your family) a nice meal. It doesn't necessarily mean you need to have concert or theater or sports event tickets every night. The goal is to do something that gives you pleasure so that you enjoy your life more than the drinking life you are leaving behind.

As I review in detail in chapter 15, one reason many people find support groups such as Alcoholics Anonymous helpful is because attending meetings helps to fill those evenings when you have nothing to do. You can learn some useful tips about how to remain abstinent while you meet other people, and it gives you a social activity that doesn't involve drinking.

DEVELOP NEW LEISURE ACTIVITIES

This is also a great time to begin some activities that you always wanted to do but didn't because drinking got in the way. Maybe you always wanted to learn how to scuba dive, take art lessons, or take a French course. Or maybe learning how to ski or play tennis or a musical instrument would be fun for you. There is a whole world out there to enjoy and there is no better time to start than now.

Why fill your time with drinking when you can have more fun doing other things? Here are more suggestions to help jump-start your thinking.

- visit a museum
- take a walk along the beach
- go to the library
- read a book
- take up a martial art
- learn to dance
- make gourmet dinners
- see a movie
- take up kickboxing
- build a piece of furniture
- enroll in a pottery class
- go parachuting

- learn to knit
- take a walk in the woods
- join a garden club
- take up astronomy
- take singing lessons
- go whitewater rafting, canoeing, or kayaking
- take up photography

If you engage in activities like these, you will have less time to think about drinking, you will have less time to drink, and you will find different life interests (and friends) that will be fun, stimulating, and exciting that don't take place in a bar and don't require that alcohol be part of the festivities.

PHYSICAL ACTIVITY

Physical activity is great for many reasons. It not only gets you in shape, it provides you with a sense of accomplishment, gives you confidence, and improves self-esteem. It is also something you can do at any time of the day, any day, to keep busy. There are many different types of physical activity from which to choose, and many you can do yourself at home. Yoga, calisthenics, running, walking, tennis, horseback riding, softball, the list is endless. Get out there and raise that pulse rate and sweat a little. It's great for the mind and the body.

You need to find the activity that feels right for you. Some people like the idea of joining a local gym, where there is a huge assortment of things to do, whether swimming, cycling, weight lifting, or running. Others prefer to work out in the privacy of their homes. Some may want to get involved in some kind of competitive team sport, whereas others may prefer a solo activity. There are a variety of outdoor and indoor activities as well. When choosing an activity, go with what interests you and see if you enjoy it. If you don't, look for something else until you find an activity that is right for you.

You also need to exercise for health reasons, but be sure to check with your doctor before you begin any exercise program. Your drinking may have taken more of a toll on you physically than you realize. You don't want to compound any problems by starting out too fast.

Aerobic Exercise Releases Endorphins

Aerobic exercise simply means any activity that uses large muscle groups and is sustained for a period of time. Aerobic exercise overloads the heart and lungs and causes them to work harder than at rest. Examples of aerobic exercise are jogging, bicycle riding, brisk walking, stair climbing, or swimming.

Aerobic exercise releases chemicals called *endorphins* in the body that are involved in fighting pain and emotional stress. Endorphins help you to maintain a good frame of mind, a state of relaxation, and a positive outlook. Endorphins can also be released through meditation.

Set Realistic Exercise Goals

Start slow. You don't want any injuries or setbacks, and you certainly don't want to discourage yourself by setting unrealistic goals. It can be hard to get started, and sometimes this can be due to having goals for yourself you can't achieve. Don't begin by setting a goal of exercising five times per week for one hour each day. Instead, start off by taking a 10-minute walk a few times each week. As you feel more inclined, you can begin to do more. Even if you are very out of shape, if you start slowly, eventually you will build up stamina and strength. But don't forget to see your doctor before starting any exercise program.

CHANGE YOUR LIFESTYLE

As you can now see, if you are going to be successful in your effort to stop drinking, you must significantly change your lifestyle so that drinking, once your favorite leisure activity, is replaced by other healthier (and more fun) activities. In addition, many of the things you liked to do while under the influence of alcohol will now have to be enjoyed without drinking alcohol—playing cards, barbecues, softball games, bowling, seeing certain friends, fishing, or even watching TV. It's quite an adjustment but entirely possible.

Keeping busy and learning to structure your day with alcohol-free activities is the best way to start, as this prevents boredom, keeps you busy, and keeps you from thinking about drinking. Over time, scheduling and doing these activities will become automatic and a part of the new, non-drinking you.

When you put your mind to it, there are many things that you can do. Enjoyable activities will strengthen your commitment to not drink, because your new life will be so satisfying and rewarding that you will not want to lose your newfound benefits.

Look around—you may also find new pleasure in things you've overlooked that are already a part of your life. For example,

— John discovered that he loved to watch his boys play hockey and eventually got involved in coaching;
— Bill developed a passion for lawn care and spent hours keeping up his yard; and
— Margaret found that she loved to experiment by cooking new and fancy meals.

DEVELOP HEALTHY PEOPLE CONNECTIONS

It is very important to have people in your life who care about you and can support your effort to achieve abstinence. It's just as important not to associate with people who will jeopardize your lifestyle change. This means that you may need to make new friends and stop associating with some old ones. When you drank, chances are you associated with others who also drank heavily. These drinking friends may even have alcohol problems themselves. As a part of your lifestyle change, you may no longer be able to see and do things with your "drinking friends."

Continuing to See Your "Drinking Friends" Is Dangerous

Let's face it. It will be extremely difficult, if not impossible, to continue to associate with your "drinking friends" and remain abstinent. Remember what I said earlier (chapter 10) about making the commitment to abstinence. As important as friends are, if abstinence is your number 1 priority, you need friends who do not have alcohol as their top priority either.

In the unlikely circumstance that you continue to see your drinking friends without it affecting your abstinence, you may no longer enjoy seeing them anyway. You will no longer have drinking in common. It is boring to sit around and watch everyone else drink and get drunk, and you'll learn that it's impossible to have a conversation of any meaning with someone who is drunk. Even fun activities aren't much fun when everyone is getting intoxicated. You'll also see how silly and stupid your good friends act when drunk. Now that you are sober, stories and antics you once thought were funny will no longer seem so cute.

Admittedly, it is not easy to cut ties with your friends. You might talk to your friends about your decision to abstain. Perhaps you can agree to see each other only when alcohol is not present, at least until you are comfortable with your decision to change your lifestyle. Seeing your friends on an individual basis as opposed to all together might be an option, as long as the friend you see agrees not to drink. If your friends cannot agree to do this, it says something about the power drinking has over them.

Reconnect with Your Friends Who Don't Drink or Who Don't Drink Heavily

You may have some friends that you lost touch with because of your drinking lifestyle, friends who can take or leave alcohol. This is an excellent time to reconnect and to re-establish friendships that were not based on drinking together. Since drinking is not the mainstay activity for these people, you may be able to socialize with them without risking a return to drinking. You can even talk to them about your decision not to drink. They will in all likelihood support your decision and encourage you to stick with it.

Developing a New Support System Takes Time

It is not easy to develop a new support system of friends and acquaintances, especially if all of your friends are heavy drinkers. If this is the case, when you first stop drinking, you will feel very lonely and disconnected, like a fish out of water. Being too isolated can lead some people to drink as much as associating with drinkers leads others to drink. This is a normal reaction, and you should anticipate it.

Coping with these feelings is another reason why many people find support groups such as Alcoholics Anonymous helpful. Attending meetings gives you an opportunity to meet new people who aren't into the drinking scene, cuts down on any feelings of isolation you may have, and helps you to develop a new support system. Without making a commitment to attend meetings forever, you may find attending meetings helpful in the short run.

Try not to get frustrated. Remember that it takes time to make new friends and change old habits. However, meeting new people and making new friendships will happen naturally in time if you keep busy, develop new interests, force yourself to explore non-drinking social opportunities, and continue to work at it.

ROMANCE

While there are no hard-and-fast rules, it is wise to avoid starting a new romantic relationship until you feel secure in your abstinence from alcohol. A new love takes your focus off of your drinking problem and can replace abstinence as your most important priority. In subtle ways, a romantic connection can take energy away from your commitment to stop drinking. You may even make some decisions based upon its effect on the new relationship, rather than weighing the outcome of those decisions on your commitment not to drink.

For example, your new love interest may want to go someplace where alcohol will be readily available. Although you know this might not be the best situation for you to be in, rather than saying no, you might go and end up drinking. Or perhaps your new lover drinks socially, and rather than refusing to drink and having to explain why you don't, you join in and begin drinking again.

Additionally, the highs and lows of a romantic encounter can be significant factors in returning to drink. If you enter into a new relationship and things do not go well, the pain and difficulties can trigger you to take "that one drink" in an effort to feel better. In short, romantic interests are complicated enough in the best of circumstances, and you do not need any added complications until you are secure in your new alcohol-free life.

While I understand that it is hard to completely avoid new love, if you do enter into a romance, remain vigilant and keep your focus on where it belongs—not drinking.

▢ ▢ ▢

There are so many things you can do in order to keep busy, pass the time, and not drink. Experiment and have fun with trying new activities, and you will find interests that you enjoy, which will help you not to drink. Eventually these activities will become a part of the new you who enjoys life even more without drinking.

Granted, it takes time for these changes to occur, but there will be a time when you don't miss drinking, don't think much about it, and thoroughly enjoy your new life even more than your former one. Use your imagination and immerse yourself in all that life has to offer. You'll never regret it.

12

MANAGING URGES TO USE

Subdue your appetites, my dears, and you've conquered human nature. CHARLES DICKENS

You may or you may not experience intense desires and urges to drink. Some people report that an urge can feel almost like a physical craving. If you do suffer from this type of urge, it's important to know that they can occur days, weeks, months, or even years after quitting, and may continue throughout your life. But that doesn't mean you should ever give into one. These urges are caused by a combination of biological, psychological, and environmental factors.

People who quit smoking also crave nicotine in the same way, as do people who used to be dependent on drugs such as painkillers or cocaine. When a person habitually uses a substance, the person's brain gets used to having it. Long after the substance has been withdrawn, there are times when the brain remembers the positive feeling it once offered. You experience this as a craving. Particularly when something in your environment reminds you of drinking, your brain can be activated and cravings can begin. Abstinence can hinge on your skill at being able to resist these kinds of urges.

MAINTAIN YOUR ENERGY LEVEL

Combating an urge to drink takes good decision making. Your "thinking brain"—responsible for controlling your behavior, reasoning things through, and taking into account any risks involved when you take action—must be sharp. When you and your thinking brain are tired, you don't think as clearly and you exercise poorer judgment. You don't want to be in that position. To be sure that "all your cells are firing," you need to get a good night's sleep. When your energy level is up, your thinking brain is strong, which helps to combat any urges to drink.

Unfortunately, sleep difficulties are quite common among people who have just stopped drinking, and they can persist for months. Problems include falling asleep, staying asleep throughout the night, and waking up earlier than usual. The first thing to keep in mind is not to be alarmed by this, since it is a common problem. Remember, too, that as uncomfortable as this is, a better sleeping pattern will return with time.

To help you get a good night's sleep, avoid drinking any caffeinated beverages in the afternoon and evening because this will only make the problem worse. Also, try not to take naps during the day, and develop a regular time when you go to bed. Over time, doing these things will help you to re-establish a better sleeping pattern.

In addition to trying to get a good night's sleep, also make sure that you aren't overdoing things and that you are getting the rest you need. Find balance in your life: if things are somewhat stressful for you and you feel drained, take time for yourself to rejuvenate, relax, and rest. Try meditating, take a bath, take a leisurely walk, or just sit down, take some deep breaths, and, as you exhale slowly, say the word *relax* to yourself. Take a break from things when you need to in order to maintain an adequate energy level.

Finally, remember to eat well, too. This is something you probably never thought much about when you used to drink, but a proper diet also helps to maintain a good energy level and decision-making abilities. A combination of carbohydrates, protein, and fat is essential. If you need help knowing what to eat, speak with your doctor, who can refer you to a nutritionist.

Heavy drinking is associated with deficiencies in many essential vitamins, including A, C, D, E, K, and B, because alcohol inhibits their absorption. Deficiencies in many minerals, such as calcium, magnesium, iron, and zinc, are quite common as well. If you don't want to see a nutritionist, at a minimum, take a daily multivitamin.

WANTING TO DRINK IS NORMAL

Wanting to drink again is normal and to be expected, even when there is nothing particularly stressful going on in your life. It is very likely (and not a sign that you are crazy) that despite all the problems alcohol has caused you, you still desire alcohol. You like to drink, and much of your drinking was enjoyable. If you didn't like to drink, you would not even be in this predicament, and like people with any other addictions who feel that they need a substance, you have a predisposition to need to drink. This is why the cravings might well pop up throughout your lifetime. So don't be surprised when you experience them. You need to accept that they are a part of staying abstinent, and you must develop ways to manage them.

KNOW WHAT TRIGGERS YOUR URGE TO DRINK

You'll notice that your urges tend to come at certain times of the day or in particular situations. This is because your drinking was linked to particular events or parts of your daily routine. Think about it: you probably drank after work, on payday, at a sporting event, with particular friends, or when you were alone. The situations that elicit your urge to drink are "triggers." Learning to identify your triggers means you can avoid these situations. If you cannot avoid triggers, you can at least plan ahead to do something different at that time.

Let's say much of your drinking occurred after work, and you notice that you begin to think about and crave alcohol as the end of the workday approaches. This means you need to change your usual routine of getting off work, going home, and making yourself a drink, and instead vary your plans. Could you go home later? Stop at the supermarket on the way?

Joe used to get home about one hour before his wife, and he struggled not to drink during this time. He decided to speak with his boss about shifting his work hours so that he could work later and arrive home right after his wife, which greatly eased his struggle and took away his urge at that time. If payday triggers your urge to drink, ensure that when you leave work, you have some plans in place that do not include drinking. Jim found that after work on payday was a difficult time for him, because all of his coworkers left to go to the local bar after work. He purposely decided to go to work later that day, so he would have to work later and wouldn't be available when everyone left to go drinking.

PAY ATTENTION TO YOUR FEELINGS

Strong negative feelings such as anger, resentment, sadness, and stress can also trigger an urge to drink. While there is never any good reason to drink, you don't want to let these feelings build up inside of you, or else you might convince yourself that you deserve a drink. Instead, you need to listen to and address your feelings.

On a daily basis, take the time to monitor how you feel and truly listen to yourself. Ask yourself if you're feeling bothered, upset, or stressed by anything. If you are, this is a sign that you need to change something in your life, and your goal is to figure out what you need to do in order to feel better. Nicole, for example, had stopped drinking for six weeks and found herself feeling so upset and stressed that she started ruminating about drinking again. She came to realize that these feelings were due to some problems she was having with her boyfriend, so instead of stuffing these feelings (or drinking over them), she talked with him, which greatly improved the relationship and helped to take away her desire to drink. Adam had a very stressful job and used to drink to deal with his feelings. After he got sober, there were times when he continued to feel stressed, and it was during these times when he began to think more about drinking. However, instead of his usual pattern of trying to ignore these feelings and drinking, he spoke with his boss, who supported his request to get some assistance. He also started to exercise after work as a way to relax.

Attending to and listening to your feelings and using them as a guide for action will feel new to you if you used to drink to cope with your feelings. Doing this will take some practice, but it will be worth the effort. Some people may find it helpful to talk with a professional therapist as they learn to deal with their emotions, which I review in chapter 16.

YOU DIDN'T QUIT BECAUSE YOU DISLIKED ALCOHOL

Remember that your decision to stop drinking had nothing to do with your no longer wanting to drink alcohol. Rather, you made the decision to quit because of all the problems your drinking caused.

I stress this point because the reason many people go back to drinking after a period of abstinence is simply because they want to. You, too, may encounter a time when you crave alcohol. If this happens to you, you can become confused about why you are not drinking, because you will choose to forget about your alcohol-related problems. Your thought process might go something like this: "I am dying for a drink . . . I want to drink . . . why shouldn't I drink? . . . it will make me feel better . . . why should I deny myself this pleasure? . . . after all, I have had a tough day (or a difficult week or month) . . . I deserve it."

Squash the urge. If you don't put a stop to this type of thinking, it is a sure bet that you will soon be drinking again. Instead, you must force yourself to remember the unpleasant ramifications and forget the pleasurable aspects of drinking.

URGES GO AWAY EVEN WITHOUT DRINKING

The good news is that *even an intense desire to drink passes*. I hear from people that if when they craved alcohol, they took their mind off it by doing something else, like going for a walk, making a phone call, or baking cookies, within a short time, like magic, the craving was gone. So, your goal must always be to get through the *momentary* and *temporary* urges to drink without drinking. The following are ways to get drinking off of your mind.

Don't Dwell on the Urge to Drink

In truth, the more you think about drinking, the more likely you are to drink, especially when you are actually experiencing a powerful urge to drink. Dwelling means continuing to think and obsess about how nice it would be to have a drink. When you begin thinking this way, you give your mind the opportunity to convince you that it is okay to have a drink. So don't dwell! Instead, get involved in some other activity, such as jogging, walking, showering, or talking to a friend. Perhaps you can go shopping or begin to read a book. Anything that can redirect your focus at the moment can help. Your goal is to get past the urge and through the moment without drinking.

Chuck found that heavy exercising seemed to help him to get past an intense urge to drink. He would go for a long jog and by the time he got back home, the urge had left him, and he didn't even want to drink anymore. Bob would immerse himself in listening to and singing along with some loud music. He would get so involved in this that he could not think about drinking, and the urge would eventually disappear. So find something that you enjoy and do it whenever the urge strikes.

Think the Drink Through

"Thinking the drink through" means forcing yourself to imagine what will happen if you start drinking again. If you have trouble getting rid of an urge, instead of actually drinking, slow things down and take the time and force yourself to remember what will happen if you drink again. Here's how:

Focus on the Harmful Consequences. When you feel the urge to drink, remind yourself of your reasons for not drinking. Those ambivalent feelings about quitting that everyone has (see chapter 3) have an uncanny way of creeping back into your mind and can begin to take over. They may push out the positive aspects of not drinking, causing you to "forget" about the harm you caused yourself when you were drinking. To combat this, read over the list you've written of harmful consequences of your drinking, and focus on this instead of taking the first drink. You should carry this list around with you at all times for quick reference in case you experience an urge and start to forget.

The Morning After. If you do give in, I guarantee that you will remember the negative consequences of your drinking *after* you take that drink. The next morning, for example, you will regret it and feel bad about doing it. Perhaps you will have a hangover or encounter the recurrence of a problem caused by the drinking. I have never heard a person who drank again after a period of abstinence say: "That was a good decision. I'm glad I drank again."

No matter how you look at it, giving into an urge to drink is a bad move and does not make your life any easier. Stay on the alcohol-free road and do what you can to not veer off of it. In the long run, this will help you achieve your goal of sobriety.

Focus on What You Don't Want to Lose. Now that you've created a fulfilling life without alcohol, you should want to keep it that way. You have worked hard, and there are people and activities in your life that you don't want to lose that bring you joy. Reminding yourself of this also helps to combat urges to drink.

JUST BECAUSE YOU *WANT* TO DRINK DOESN'T MEAN YOU SHOULD—EVER!

I want to share one of my favorite mantras with you in the hope that you'll practice saying it to yourself: "Of course, I want to drink. However, I can choose not to because I don't want to deal with the consequences that have resulted and will result from my drinking." When you feel the desire to drink, repeat this. Over time, this mantra, along with the other advice in this chapter, should help you to develop confidence that you can successfully handle urges.

Remember, too, that you have a choice between drinking and not drinking. For some, the idea that they *can't* ever drink again bothers them tremendously. To fight this, they tell themselves, "Who says I can't drink?" However, when they remember that they *can* drink, but that they *choose* not to, they feel comforted. Of course, you can drink again if you want to drink. You are simply choosing not to do that for the day, because your life is better when you don't consume alcohol.

REACH OUT FOR SUPPORT

It can be particularly helpful to talk about your intense urge with someone who knows you are trying to stop and with whom you feel comfortable. This person should also be available when you need to talk. This person may be your partner, spouse, sibling, parent, or friend. It doesn't matter. What does matter is their willingness to help and your respect for their opinion of you. Scott discovered that whenever he felt like drinking, calling his wife Sandy and talking with her about how he was feeling always helped him to get past his urge. He stated: "After I speak with her and tell her that I won't drink, I just can't. I don't know if it's that I can't let her down or me down, but the decision is made and then I just do something else until I see her. And once I see her, I know the battle is over."

Making the effort to talk with someone about your urge to drink can often take the urge away. Make sure this person can remind you about the reasons why you are not drinking, which you will need to hear to overcome your urge to drink.

⬜ ⬜ ⬜

Overcoming the urge to drink is an important skill and one you'll need to master so you can quit drinking successfully. The good news is that there are many ways to handle urges and remain sober. And believe me—over time you will get better and better at doing this, and urges will come less often and will usually be less intense. Remembering the following will help you to handle your urges:

- Wanting to drink is normal and to be expected.
- Urges can and do go away without drinking.
- Figure out what your triggers are and avoid them, or make changes in your life to decrease your desire to drink.
- Distract yourself and don't dwell on the urge.
- Think through the urge by focusing on the negative consequences of drinking and what you will lose if you drink.
- Remember that there will always be times when you want to drink . . . but that you can choose not to drink.
- Reach out for support.

13

SLIPS AND FALLS ON THE PATH TO SOBRIETY

Just keep going. Everybody gets better if they keep at it.
TED WILLIAMS

A person who is trying to stay abstinent, especially a newly sober person, will often slip (lapse) or fall (relapse). A slip or lapse is when a person temporarily returns to drinking for a short period of time and doesn't suffer major consequences as a result. A fall or relapse implies a heavy involvement with alcohol after a period of abstinence, and in all likelihood, bigger alcohol-related problems. When trying to stay abstinent, any drinking is a very serious matter, signaling that you are not in control and that trouble is just around the corner. Obviously, the more lapses you have, the greater the chance that a relapse will eventually take place.

Especially when you first stop drinking, as you achieve success you can grow confident, even cocky, and the structure and careful decision making that enabled you to stop drinking can erode. For example, you may resume previously avoided activities where alcohol is available, or you may begin to reconnect with friends who drink heavily. You might think that you can handle these situations but find yourself drinking again within a fairly short time.

To succeed, you need to maintain your focus on not drinking. Especially in the early months, you can't allow overconfidence to get in the way. Don't let down your guard. Staying sober still needs to be your top priority.

In this chapter, I will outline the three most common traps that will challenge your sobriety after a period of abstinence. Knowing about them will prevent a lapse or relapse. If you do lapse or relapse, this chapter will also help you to understand what happened so you can be on guard for this in the future. But first, a few words about managing a lapse or relapse if it occurs.

MANAGING LAPSES AND RELAPSES

While a lapse in not drinking is real, it does not have to result in a full-blown serious relapse. The quicker you end your lapse, the less harm it will cause to your future sobriety. If you have a lapse or even a relapse, minimize the harm. If you take a drink, it doesn't need to escalate into a relapse. For instance, if you take a drink, rather than saying "Well, there's nothing I can do about it now, so I might as well really get drunk," instead say to yourself, "I drank, but I must stop now and prevent further harm to myself." Or let's assume you had a few drinks one evening. Instead of saying, "Well I screwed up my sobriety so I might as well drink tonight, too," say "Okay, I drank before, but I don't have to do it again."

Don't view a lapse or relapse as a personal failure, don't beat yourself up, and attempt to learn from it. A lapse or relapse can help you see where the holes are in your recovery program and what you need to work on to prevent a future slip. If you get really down on yourself for drinking again, your self-blame could lead to further drinking as a way to deal with the pain of "failure." Finding fault with yourself does nothing positive for you and takes your attention away from your number 1 priority: abstinence.

Don't Discount Your Sobriety, but Don't Discount the Lapse

It is also important to remember that a lapse or relapse does not destroy your past period of abstinence. If you were abstinent for two months and relapsed, or were abstinent for two years and relapsed, this is certainly better than if you had been continuously drinking throughout this time. Drinking again, while a serious concern, does not mean that you start back at the beginning. Feel positive about having been abstinent for that period of time.

On the other hand, don't minimize what has happened. Drinking again needs to be taken seriously. You will need to understand what played a role in your return to drinking. By doing this, you will better understand what you need to do differently in order to achieve success.

Learn, Learn, Learn

If you return to drinking, think about what circumstances and events in your life precipitated your lapse. Life moves quickly, and we're often too busy to look closely at the factors that play a role in our decision making. But this is exactly what you need to do to better understand yourself.

Try thinking of your life as a movie. Slow the movie down and look at it frame by frame. In one frame, you may not be thinking about drinking. In the next, you may have begun to think about it or actually started drinking. Review that micro-moment in extreme detail to see what was happening in your life and within your mind. Were you bored or lonely? Were you with people who were triggers for you or were you in a drinking situation that was risky? Perhaps you were feeling particularly stressed. By looking back in detail, you can learn what precipitated your slip and what you need to do differently to prevent this from happening again.

Dave, a 52-year-old man, had stopped drinking successfully for about four months. To his dismay, found himself drinking again, which again caused him problems. He couldn't understand why he started drinking again, as his life had been going so much better since he had decided to stop. When he closely examined the circumstances of his relapse, he discovered that being away on business alone was the trigger. He realized that when he was alone at night with nothing to do, he began to ruminate about drinking, and eventually he began to drink. During those times, he also convinced himself that "no one would know anyway," and that if he drank away from home, it "didn't really matter."

As a way to better cope with this situation, Dave learned to carefully structure his evenings when away on business and to plan activities after work that did not include being around alcohol. He also learned not to allow his thinking to trick him into believing that it was fine to drink away from home. This insight and change in his behavior enabled him to avoid drinking in these situations, and he successfully achieved abstinence again.

Like any new activity or endeavor, be it playing tennis, skiing, working on a computer, or golf, success at refraining from drinking depends on learning and developing skills. Basic skills come first and then, over time, more refined skills are acquired. As we practice, we get better and better at whatever task we are attempting, including the task of not drinking. If you drink again, the important point is to learn from the experience and to discover what you need to do differently to not drink in the future. The key is to learn from your mistakes so that you don't repeat the same ones over and over again.

THE THREE COMMON TRAPS

For more than 20 years, I have worked with people who struggle with their use of alcohol, and I've learned a lot about how people convince themselves to pick up a drink after having made the decision to no longer do this. While sometimes this happens because they simply didn't foresee a potential problem (they ended up in a situation where everyone was drinking and before they knew it, they drank, too), more often, it has to do with other factors. What is so amazing is that they often know these things, but at the moment they "forget" or don't think about them.

In the last three chapters, I reviewed a number of techniques and strategies you need to incorporate into your daily life so that you can achieve abstinence. I consider them to be the basics and essential to carry out and remember for you to be successful. Although you read them, you, too, may "forget" about some of them, which can cause you to lapse or relapse. You also may not have fully integrated some of these strategies, and this can play a role in your returning to drinking. So I will review some of those ideas for you now. There is a big difference between being exposed to skills and mastering them. The goal here is to re-expose you to some of these critical skills so that you can achieve mastery.

You need to be on guard for three main traps if you are going to stay on the path of sobriety. Knowing these traps will help prevent your returning to drinking and shed light on what is responsible for your setback, if you have one.

1. Wanting to Drink and "Forgetting" the Consequences

Let's face it—you like the feeling of intoxication, and this contributed to your problem of drinking excessively. When you finally decided to stop drinking, it wasn't because you suddenly disliked alcohol, but because drinking too much was causing you problems. You were sick and tired of the social, financial, legal, health-related, and other problems brought on by consuming too much alcohol. However, the fondness for the feeling that intoxication brings you is another reason why it's difficult to follow a path of sobriety. That feeling of being high is hard to give up and often comes back to haunt you.

As I reviewed in the last chapter, there are going to be times when you'll crave a drink. I offered many ways for you to deal with this feeling, whether by not dwelling on it and pushing it out of your mind, distracting yourself, or thinking the desire through and re-membering the harmful consequences of your drinking. Despite knowing these techniques, many people return to alcohol simply because they *want to drink*.

Some of my research has involved a questionnaire that asks people who struggle with alcohol if they have ever relapsed, and if so, what was responsible. The questionnaire contained about 35 different reasons for relapse, and people were asked to identify the most impor-tant factors in their relapse. Of all of the reasons, one of the most common was *wanting to drink*.

If you had a lapse or relapse and wanting to drink was a factor, go back and reread the last chapter on how to manage urges to drink.

Learning to successfully resist a desire to drink and getting past that momentary feeling is essential. And let me again share with you one of my favorite mantras: "Of course, I want to drink. However, I can choose not to because I don't want to deal with the consequences that resulted and will result from my drinking." *You must force yourself to think the drink through and remember all of the harmful consequences that resulted from your drinking.*

Figure Out Why You Want to Drink. You should also consider why you want to drink so much. While the feeling of wanting to drink is normal for anyone who has had an alcohol problem, you may also experience a strong desire to drink because alcohol fills an important need. Think about why drinking is so important to you. Is there is something missing in your life now that alcohol is no longer there? Do you feel a void? If you can understand what alcohol fulfills for you, you can learn ways to meet those needs, your desire to drink will lessen, and you'll grow as a person.

Jerry is a 38-year-old, single man who decided to abstain because he could no longer deal with hangovers and missing work. He stopped drinking for two months, but due to wanting to drink, he relapsed and started missing work again.

Jerry began looking at himself to understand why he craved alcohol. He found that without alcohol, he didn't know how to have a good time with others. Alcohol was his social lubricant and lessened his self-consciousness and anxiety. When he stopped drinking, he also stopped socializing and began to feel more and more isolated.

Jerry began experimenting with other alcohol-free social activities and forced himself to confront his anxiety. As he learned to have fun without drinking and to better manage his anxiety, his desire to drink decreased.

Understandably, this may be difficult for some of you to do on your own, especially if your anxiety is severe. In that case, you may need extra help to better manage these feelings. Seeing a professional therapist can enable you to develop the skills to do this, which I review in chapter 16.

Try to discover why you like to drink so much. If you can, direct your efforts to satisfy those needs in other ways, which will decrease some of your strong feelings to drink.

2. Believing You Can Control Your Drinking

Now wait a minute. How can the thought that you can control your drinking be responsible for a lapse or a relapse? After all, you may have already learned that you can't do this because you tried to moderate your drinking, weren't able to, and then chose to stop drinking entirely. Or you knew right off the bat that you couldn't learn to moderate your drinking, and without having to prove this to yourself, decided on abstinence. In chapter 10, I reviewed the idea that abstinence is abstinence forever, and that for you, moderating drinking is impossible. How can you forget this, when forgetting allows you to decide to pick up a drink? Your mind has an amazing ability to forget the fact that you can't moderate your drinking. This forgetting is called denial. While you may have understood that you could not drink at all when you first began your path to sobriety, over time this thought often melts away and evaporates. What seemed so clear at the beginning becomes less so.

Denial. While in the strict sense, denial refers to a person's failure even to acknowledge an alcohol problem, in a broader context denial includes the minimization of a drinking problem, such as believing that one drink is acceptable. Acknowledging that alcohol is a problem but believing that it can be controlled, when it cannot, is also a form of denial. This form sabotages sobriety and is a much more common and typical variety of denial than is not believing that you even have an alcohol problem. You must guard against it.

Perhaps you have said one of the following things to yourself:

- "I have a problem, but I'm not that bad!"
- "Sure, I have an alcohol problem, but I can drink occasionally if I'm careful."
- "One drink won't hurt!"
- "I can control my drinking most of the time."
- "I've been clean for 2 months . . . I can have one or two drinks."

Sound like you? If you tell yourself that your problem isn't that bad, or that you can control your use of alcohol, even some of time, or that it is okay to have one drink, you will eventually drink again. This same scenario occurs with other behaviors. Remember the Lay's potato chip commercial slogan: "Bet you can't eat just one"? Well, most people couldn't. One chip turned into too many. And the same happens with smokers or problem gamblers.

How often have you known friends who quit smoking and then one day, decide to have a cigarette, *just one cigarette?* Before long, they are buying a pack. At the moment they had the first cigarette, they knew that cigarette smoking was a problem for them, but they convinced themselves that it would be fine to have just one. They never believed that having just one cigarette would lead them to full-blown smoking again. They denied that fact that they couldn't moderate their smoking.

Your Love of Drinking Causes Denial. The major factor that creates denial or allows you to minimize your drinking problem is that you love to drink. You don't want to admit that you can't drink at all, because you enjoy drinking. So, in order to continue to drink, you tell yourself that your drinking isn't that bad or that you can control it.

In fact, if you didn't love drinking, denial would never be an issue. You would simply acknowledge that alcohol causes you problems, and you would stop drinking. After all, who wants to continue to do something which creates trouble? It is your love of alcohol and the wish to continue to drink that fuels the denial.

Overcoming Denial. Reread pages 134–35 in chapter 10. Those pages contain critical information that will help you avoid the trap of believing that you can moderate your drinking or even have one drink. Also review the written list of harmful consequences related to your drinking suggested on pages 133–34. This will help you to remember how bad your drinking really was and that you truly can't drink. You should also reread the cons of your drinking in the *Pros and Cons of My Drinking* exercise that you completed in chapter 3. Doing this will keep your focus on the seriousness of your drinking problem and what happens when you drink.

Finally, write down all of the times you unsuccessfully tried to limit your drinking and the times you planned to have just one drink (or a few) and, instead, drank to excess. I am sure there are many times you did this, and writing them down and forcing yourself to admit this helps to counter the power of denial.

Thinking that drinking can be safely controlled and that one or two drinks will not lead to more is an extremely common trap. *You must be on guard for this type of thinking.* Remember that this thinking is just your mind playing a trick on you. Knowing this will prevent you from falling for it.

3. Painful Feelings

Experiencing painful feelings is another big trigger that can lead you to break your sobriety and return to drinking. It is no wonder this happens. Throughout your life, you have learned to use alcohol as a way to cope. For example, after having a stressful day at work, you used alcohol in order to relax. After a conflict with a loved one, alcohol eased your stress. If you felt anxious or worried about something, alcohol was there. A relationship breaks up? Use alcohol. And the list goes on and on.

When feeling upset, your usual and customary way of coping was using alcohol. After years of doing this, your painful feelings and your use of alcohol got linked together. So now, when you experience any of these feelings, your desire to drink increases.

In chapter 10, you learned that there is never a good reason to drink, and that regardless of what you feel, drinking isn't the answer. In fact, drinking will make everything worse. But when you feel pain, what can you do instead?

Sit with Your Feelings. First, learn to "sit with your feelings" and realize that you don't need to rid yourself of your painful feelings immediately. Learn to be more comfortable with feeling bad, which can be quite an adjustment for you. This is an important point, because I bet you probably used alcohol as a "quick fix" to manage your discomfort. Whenever you felt bad, you drank, which at least temporarily took away your pain. As a result, now when you aren't drinking, you aren't comfortable sitting with your feelings. Get to know your feelings and don't be afraid of them.

Painful Feelings Get Better in Time. Understand that painful feelings often go away, or at least get better, within a fairly short period of time without your doing anything. What seems overwhelming at the moment often gets easier all on its own. I'm sure that you probably don't know this, because you never gave yourself the opportunity to discover it. You drank, and if you felt better, you thought it was due to the alcohol. In reality, the alcohol may have had little, if anything, to do with it. Take Mary, for instance. She used to get very upset and stressed at work and drank after work to cope. When she first stopped drinking, she was concerned about how she was going to deal with her stress. But what Mary found, much to her surprise, was that after a few hours, even if she didn't drink, she began to feel more relaxed. For her, it was an amazing insight.

But be patient. Sometimes it takes more than a few hours to feel better. For example, you're not going to get over a relationship breakup over night. However, you will get over it in time. Remember the one-day-at-a-time philosophy I reviewed in chapter 10. Just get through the day, which is all you need to do.

Try to Understand Your Feelings. Getting to know your feelings also gives you insight into yourself and what you need to do differently to feel better. For example, maybe you find that your pain consists of holding in anger and stress due to a conflict you are having. If this fits for you, you need to express these feelings directly and face the conflict head on. If you find this difficult, there are numerous books that can help you to become more assertive and be better able to deal with conflict. These can be found in most bookstores by looking for books that have the word *assertiveness* in their titles. Or you could log onto www.amazon .com and type in the word *assertiveness,* and you will be able to peruse these kinds of books. Seeing a professional therapist could also be helpful for this kind of problem if you think you need extra help.

If you're feeling stressed about something you can't change at the moment, remember that there are other ways to manage things besides drinking. Deep breathing, walking, exercising, talking to a friend, or reading can be very useful to help manage your feelings and enable you to get through the difficult time. There are again numerous books that can teach you to better manage stress in your life, and, again, these can be found in most bookstores or by logging onto www.amazon.com. The key words to look for or type in order to find these kinds of books are *stress management, meditation,* and *relaxation training.*

Common painful feelings in early recovery are boredom and loneliness, which can be uncomfortable and troubling. In fact, my research has shown that these feelings are some of the most common reasons for relapse. And it is no wonder that these feelings often trigger a return to drinking— you are now trying to develop a new lifestyle that may include finding new friends, a new support system, new interests, and new leisure activities. And developing a new lifestyle can be a frustrating process that takes time.

Chapter 11 reviewed how you need to change your lifestyle and fill the void left by alcohol. You don't want a lot of idle time on your hands, and you don't want to be a "dry drunk." If you are experiencing loneliness and boredom, it is a sign that you need to place a greater emphasis on creating a fulfilling life for yourself without alcohol. Let your imagination go wild and force yourself to think of fun things you can do.

SOMETIMES YOU MIGHT NEED HELP

There are people who, in addition to their alcohol problem, struggle with a psychiatric disorder, such as severe feelings of depression or anxiety. Others may suffer from a terrible self-concept, poor self-esteem, or have trouble in developing meaningful relationships with others. If this describes you, know that there is help available, which I will review in the next section of this book. Remember that even in these situations, drinking isn't the answer. It will just make everything worse.

▯ ▯ ▯

So those are the three big traps that can get you off track and lead you back to drinking. While you know that these aren't reasons to drink (in fact, there are no reasons to drink), these traps have an insidious way of sneaking up on you. It's easy to get fooled, and you can "forget" why you stopped drinking in the first place.

Remembering these common traps will help prevent you from picking up that first drink and will decrease the chance of your drinking again. And if you did lapse or relapse, knowing these will help you understand what happened and will enable you to avoid a relapse in the future.

PART V
OTHER RESOURCES

14

THE NEED FOR
OUTSIDE TREATMENT

There is no failure except in no longer trying.

ELBERT HUBBARD

In spite of your best efforts and hard work, you may continue to experience problems related to drinking and you may need to seek outside help. How do you know for sure if you fall into this category? If any of the statements below describe you, it is likely you need help if you want to live a sober and happy life:

- You are not able to maintain abstinence for any significant period of time.
- You are able to achieve abstinence but occasionally relapse, with a return of drinking-related problems.
- You're unable to moderate your drinking and still will not consider abstinence, even though your life is full of alcohol-related difficulties.
- You have achieved abstinence, but you are not enjoying life.

- You have come to the conclusion that you need help to remain sober, but aren't sure where to turn.

Any of these predicaments can be daunting and overwhelming. Who do you turn to and where can you get the help that you need? You may have no idea what help is available and literally don't know where to begin. Or maybe you've heard of AA, but aren't sure if it's for you, and have no information about other kinds of available help.

On the other hand, you may have heard of all different kinds of treatment options—from hospitals, to rehabs, to outpatient programs, to halfway houses, to a range of self-help groups—but you don't know what's best for you, and you're confused about what to do next. Add to this all of the different types of therapists you may have heard of, such as psychologists, psychiatrists, social workers, and alcohol counselors, and your confusion can be even further magnified.

In today's world, with so many treatment options, you need to be an educated consumer. You want to get the right treatment the first time rather than getting involved in the wrong program, or seeing the wrong therapist, and wasting your time. The good news is that ensuring you get the best help is not as complicated as it sounds, and you can learn how to do it. But first, a few words about your decision to seek help.

DON'T BE UPSET WITH YOURSELF

You've tried hard to help yourself, and although you may have had some success, things still aren't where you want them. You may be thinking, "What is wrong with me?" or "Why can't I get it?" You may feel like a failure for being unable to help yourself with your problem, and that's a terrible place to be.

Try not to beat yourself up because you need some additional support. Finding yourself a little stuck at times is human nature. The problem with getting a handle on your drinking may have absolutely nothing to do with your individual effort or the lack of it; difficulties occur for reasons that aren't in your control. In many cases, an outside observer can help you to look at your situation in a different way and, with a new perspective, you'll succeed by trying a different route. Who cares if you need some help? The most important thing is that you're trying to help yourself and you're not giving up.

Don't let shame or embarrassment get in the way either. These feelings can stop you from getting the help you need. Even if you make it to your first appointment, they can get in the way of your being totally honest. You have nothing to be ashamed or embarrassed about. You have a drinking problem, and that's it. Think back to chapter 2, when you learned why you may have a drinking problem. It has nothing to do with your character. You're just stuck in a certain way of being in the world, like we all get at some point in our lives.

SEEKING OUTSIDE HELP IS A POSITIVE MOVE

Taking control of your drinking problem is what this book is all about. Whether you're able to do this without any help other than reading this book, or you need a little outside assistance, the critical and most important thing is that you are addressing your problem with alcohol. Your willingness to actively seek help demonstrates your commitment to getting better. That's something to be proud of.

In the next three chapters, you'll learn about the various types of treatment options available for you. Almost all of these options maintain that abstinence is the only way to recover from a drinking problem. The only exceptions are the Moderation Management self-help program and meeting with a therapist privately, which could have moderate drinking as your goal of treatment. There may also be some professional therapy groups that have this as a treatment goal as well.

You'll discover that some of these treatment programs are highly structured and are indicated if you have been having a lot of difficulty resolving your drinking problem—for example, if you have not been able to put together any significant periods of sobriety and your drinking is still causing you major problems. Others are less structured and are more appropriate if you have been able to achieve some success but still have problems caused by your drinking. If you find that less structured treatment isn't helping you, you'll need more intensive treatment. If you continue to experience problems with alcohol consumption, even with treatment, abstinence *must* be your route to recovery.

15

SELF-HELP GROUPS

Man is a social animal.   BARUCH SPINOZA

Self-help groups are outside of the formalized, professional alcoholism-treatment system. In fact, self-help groups have been developed by people who struggled with drinking and were not getting the help they needed through professional treatment. In addition, these programs are free!

The first self-help program specifically designed to help those who struggle with alcohol was Alcoholics Anonymous, or AA. Other self-help programs have been developed for the same purpose. These other programs were started because different things work with different people, and AA wasn't working for some people. Some found that AA wasn't a good match for them due to philosophical differences regarding how to understand and help a person who has a drinking problem.

Many people find self-help groups invaluable. Because you are surrounded with people who also struggle with alcohol, self-help groups can provide you with a place where you are accepted for who you are. If you're feeling bad about yourself, this warm environment can help you feel better. Also, if your present situation is very bad, being around others who have "been there" and have "gotten through it" can be wonderful and can help you remember that there is hope and that you, too, will get through it. Being around others who struggle with the same problem as you do can also help to reduce the destructive "me-against-the-world" feeling that you might have, as you'll find firsthand that there are many, many people in your situation.

Self-help groups can also provide you with a new social support system, which can be critically important, especially if most people in your life drink. Remember that if you are going to stop drinking, you can't continue to associate with your drinking friends and be surrounded by alcohol. In addition, if you have lost many significant relationships because of your drinking, you'll have the opportunity to develop new friendships, which can help to make up for these losses and the void you may feel. And you will meet people who don't, or are at least trying not to, drink.

Attending meetings can also give you something to do with your time. As mentioned before, loneliness and boredom are often huge concerns, particularly when you first stop drinking. There will also be times when you simply don't know what to do with yourself, and you'll feel like you have an awful lot of time on your hands. Knowing that you'll be attending a meeting helps structure your day, gives you something to do, and helps with boredom and loneliness.

The most prominent self-help groups in the United States are Alcoholics Anonymous (AA), Moderation Management (MM), Secular

Organizations for Sobriety (SOS), SMART Recovery, and Women for Sobriety (WFS). Except for MM, all of these programs maintain that you must achieve abstinence to resolve your drinking problem. I will also review Rational Recovery (RR), which used to be a self-help group but is now a self-help resource. RR also insists on abstinence.

All of these programs have their own philosophies and ways of offering help; the key is to find one that fits with your own belief system. For some, AA has been an absolute lifesaver and the essential ingredient in resolving their drinking problem. Others have found that the philosophy of AA rubbed them wrong. They could never connect to that program and found much more benefit through another program. When looking for a self-help program, listen to your feelings and make the choice that's right for you.

In what follows, you'll learn about each of these programs and their basic philosophy and approach, and this will help to steer you in the right direction. However, I encourage you to shop around, as there is nothing like experiencing a meeting firsthand to know whether it's right for you.

ALCOHOLICS ANONYMOUS

Almost everyone has heard of AA, which is the best-known self-help recovery program in the world. AA has an estimated more than two million members throughout the world, with about half of them in the United States, and there are more than 100,000 AA groups. Since AA first came into existence, many other self-help groups have been modeled after it to help people who suffer from different addictions, including Narcotics Anonymous, Cocaine Anonymous, Pills Anonymous, Gamblers Anonymous, Debtors Anonymous, and Overeaters Anonymous.

AA was first developed in 1935 by Bill W. and Dr. Bob, both of whom were alcoholic. They began talking to each other, which helped Dr. Bob to stop drinking (Bill W. was already abstinent), and soon after, both men began working with other people who struggled with alcohol. A few groups of alcoholics talking with other alcoholics began to meet, and four years later, AA published its basic textbook, *Alcoholics Anonymous.*

The Program

AA encourages complete and total abstinence from alcohol. It believes that alcoholism is a disease and that recovery is a life-long process. When people speak at meetings, they always mention their first name and the fact that they are an alcoholic or addict. When you first start attending meetings, however, if you don't feel comfortable introducing yourself as an alcoholic, you don't have to do this. AA suggests that recovery from an alcohol problem can only be accomplished "one day at a time" by following the Twelve Steps of AA, the first of which is to admit powerlessness over alcohol. A strong emphasis is placed on a "Higher Power," however you choose to understand this, outside of yourself to help you refrain from drinking. While AA is not a religious organization, it has a strong spiritual component.

There are different types of AA meetings, including speaker meetings, discussion meetings, step meetings in which the Twelve Steps of AA are discussed, and meetings for beginners, which often meet before a larger meeting. Meetings can be open to anyone or open only to those who have a desire to stop drinking. There are also more specialized groups for women, men, young people, and gay people. Groups vary in size from just a few members to hundreds of members.

THE TWELVE STEPS OF ALCOHOLICS ANONYMOUS

1. We admitted we were powerless over alcohol—that our lives had become unmanageable.
2. Came to believe that a power greater than ourselves could restore us to sanity.
3. Made a decision to turn our will and our lives over to the care of God *as we understood Him.*
4. Made a searching and fearless moral inventory of ourselves.
5. Admitted to God, to ourselves, and to another human being the exact nature of our wrongs.
6. Were entirely ready to have God remove all these defects of character.
7. Humbly asked Him to remove our shortcomings.
8. Made a list of all persons we had harmed, and became willing to make amends to them all.
9. Made direct amends to such people wherever possible, except when to do so would injure them or others.
10. Continued to take personal inventory and when we were wrong promptly admitted it.
11. Sought through prayer and meditation to improve our conscious contact with God *as we understood Him,* praying only for knowledge of His will for us and the power to carry that out.
12. Having had a spiritual awakening as a result of these steps, we tried to carry this message to alcoholics and to practice these principles in all our affairs.

In speaker meetings, members who have maintained abstinence tell their story. Speakers talk about when they first used alcohol, when and how their alcohol use became destructive, and, finally, their own salvation through abstinence and their involvement in the program of AA. Other members identify with aspects of these stories, which provide a model for their own recovery. There are also speaker discussion meetings, when a discussion takes place after the speakers have told their stories.

Discussion meetings generally focus on a particular aspect of the recovery process. These can be open to anyone or "closed" (open only to those who have a desire to stop drinking). Discussion meetings provide members the opportunity to discuss different aspects and phases of their alcohol problem. Discussion meetings can be particularly helpful to newer members, who can direct their questions to longer-standing members who have a wealth of personal experience. "Beginners'" meetings are specifically for those who are just beginning AA, who have been sober for a shorter period of time, or who are returning to the program after a lapse or relapse.

In step meetings, participants discuss particular steps of the program. The steps are essentially a group of principles, spiritual in nature, which, if followed, can rid the alcoholic of the obsession to drink and help the person to become happy and fulfilled.

Another important aspect to the program is the use of a sponsor of your choice, who is another AA member in solid recovery. AA suggests a sponsor of the same sex to decrease the chances of any emotional distractions. By providing guidance and support, the sponsor can be a key individual in your recovery. Often a sponsor is readily available to talk by telephone and can meet you at or take you to meetings.

At meetings, you may hear about the absolute devastation someone has experienced due to drinking, and this could make you think that you aren't "bad enough" to go to AA. Don't worry. The philosophy of AA is to identify with what you can and to forget the rest, which is good advice. AA uses the expression, "There but for the grace of God go I." This means that whatever you hear could possibly describe you, perhaps not in your current state, but at some point in the future. There are certainly people who, at an earlier time in their lives, could not believe the damage that alcohol would eventually cause them. When they first attended AA meetings and heard others tell their stories, they said that that would never happen to them. Years later, however, their lives were even worse. Don't allow the feeling that you're not as bad as others prevent you from getting help.

For some, attending AA meetings becomes a way of life, and AA eventually becomes a very important part of their identity. They may even go on "commitments," when they volunteer to speak at other AA meetings as a way to help other alcoholics. For others, AA is a once or twice a week meeting that helps them, and that is all they need. Many people attend meetings very often in the beginning, when they need more support to stay abstinent, and less frequently after they have been sober for many months or years. While AA suggests that AA should become a way of life, it is certainly fine to use it in a way that feels right for you.

If you decide to go to AA and eventually want to stop going to meetings, you may hear that you are headed for a relapse. Certainly, some people have dropped out of AA and relapsed, but others have remained sober. Everyone is different, and no one approach is right for everyone. While some may need to remain in AA to successfully recover from their drinking problems, others may benefit from a more limited involvement in terms of the frequency of attendance, commitment to AA, and the length of time one attends meetings.

Finding Out More

AA has many meetings, and you are almost sure to find one near where you live, so a good way to learn about AA is to attend the meetings. Go to at least two or three per week for a couple of months. Don't be put off if you don't like your first meeting. Every meeting has its own character and size. Check out some different meetings until you find the ones that make you feel comfortable. Remember that the mix of individuals is different in each group, and some groups will feel better to you than others.

Another excellent way to learn about AA is to talk to someone who is in the program. He or she would probably be happy to bring you to a meeting. To find out where meetings are held, check your local telephone directory for a listing for Alcoholics Anonymous or call their main number at (212) 870-3400. The AA office can tell you where meetings are held in your area, and they will send you a meeting booklet. For more information, write to AA at: Grand Central Station, Box 459, New York, NY 10163. A wealth of information also is available at their website, www.alcoholics-anonymous.org. I would also suggest two of their publications: *Alcoholics Anonymous* (known in AA as "the Big Book") and *Twelve Steps and Twelve Traditions*.

MODERATION MANAGEMENT

Moderation Management (MM) was founded by Audrey Kishline in 1993, when she realized that there were no support groups for people who had problems with alcohol and wanted to try to moderate their drinking. She had struggled with drinking herself and received abstinence-oriented treatment, which she didn't find helpful. Over time, she began to moderate her drinking, and eventually she developed the MM program. As you'll learn, the underlying philosophy of MM is similar to my own and to what I have outlined in this book, and it is the one self-help program that supports the goal of moderate drinking.

You may have heard that seven years after founding MM, Ms. Kishline killed two people in a car accident. She was intoxicated at the time, was arrested for drunk driving, and was sent to jail. At her trial, her lawyer said, "The accident and the subsequent intensive alcohol treatment she has undergone have made Kishline realize that moderation management is nothing but alcoholics covering up their problem."

While I do not know the motivation behind this statement, regardless of Ms. Kishline's difficulties, it is clear that some people who have struggled with alcohol are able to learn how to moderate their drinking so that alcohol no longer causes them problems. In chapters 2 and 6, I reviewed this concept and noted that, while some can learn to control drinking, not everyone can. Because Ms. Kishline could not learn to control her drinking does not mean that no one can be successful with this approach.

Using this kind of logic would mean that if one person could not learn to achieve abstinence, then no one could, which is not true. Or that if a person achieved abstinence by attending AA meetings, and years later relapsed, then AA and its focus on abstinence should be seen as a misguided and flawed program. Obviously, this makes no sense. What does make sense is that alcohol problems are very complicated and that there are a variety of strategies that people can use to stop alcohol from ruining their lives, including learning how to moderate their drinking.

MM's NINE STEPS TOWARD MODERATION AND POSITIVE LIFESTYLE CHANGES

1. Attend meetings or online groups and learn about the program of Moderation Management.
2. Abstain from alcoholic beverages for 30 days and complete steps three through six during this time.
3. Examine how drinking has affected your life.
4. Write down your life priorities.
5. Take a look at how much, how often, and under what circumstances you had been drinking.
6. Learn the MM guidelines and limits for moderate drinking.
7. Set moderate drinking limits and start weekly "small steps" toward balance and moderation in other areas of your life.
8. Review your progress and update your goals.
9. Continue to make positive lifestyle changes and attend meetings whenever you need ongoing support or would like to help others.

The Program

Moderation Management (MM) is a behavioral-change support program for people who are concerned about their drinking. MM maintains that alcohol problems can vary from moderate to severe, and that people should be free to choose their own goal about how to resolve their drinking problem, whether by abstinence or moderation. MM states that it is best for a person to address a drinking problem early, before it becomes more severe. MM also acknowledges that people who have serious alcohol problems will probably need to resolve their drinking problem via abstinence, but at the same time, MM maintains that such people need to figure this out for themselves.

MM offers nine steps toward moderation and positive lifestyle changes, and also gives recommendations about how much a person should drink.

Finding Out More

For more information about MM, you can call (212) 871-0974. Their website, www.moderation.org, contains a lot of information about the program including where meetings are held. There aren't a lot of MM meetings, but MM maintains an active online community where members can get support. The book to read to learn more about MM is *Moderate Drinking: The Moderation Management Guide for People Who Want to Reduce Their Drinking,* by Audrey Kishline.

SECULAR ORGANIZATIONS FOR SOBRIETY

Secular Organizations for Sobriety (SOS), informally known as "Save Our Selves," was formed in 1985 by Jim Christopher, who wrote an article about achieving sobriety through personal responsibility and self-reliance. After receiving an overwhelming response to this article, he eventually founded the organization.

The Program

SOS is a nonreligious support group for people who want to learn how to quit using alcohol or other drugs. It is an alternative to AA because it does not emphasize spiritual or religious beliefs. Meetings don't focus on religion or spirituality; SOS believes that an alcohol problem is a separate, nonreligious issue. People don't need to be agnostic or atheist to attend. Anyone of any religious orientation is welcome.

SOS emphasizes the importance of self-empowerment to achieve abstinence and suggests that to be successful, no longer drinking must be the "Priority One, no matter what!"

SOS SUGGESTED GUIDELINES FOR SOBRIETY

To break the cycle of denial and achieve sobriety, we first acknowledge that we are alcoholics or addicts.

We reaffirm this truth daily and accept without reservation the fact that as clean and sober individuals, we cannot and do not drink or use, no matter what.

Since drinking or using is not an option for us, we take whatever steps are necessary to continue our Sobriety Priority lifelong.

A quality of life, "the good life," can be achieved. However, life is also filled with uncertainties. Therefore, we do not drink or use regardless of feelings, circumstances, or conflicts.

We share in confidence with each other our thoughts and feelings as sober, clean individuals.

Sobriety is our Priority, and we are each responsible for our lives and sobriety.

Source: James Christopher, *How to Stay Sober: Recovery without Religion* (Prometheus Books 1988).

SOS meetings usually are attended by about 12 people and are generally loose and informal. A chairperson often comes up with a topic to discuss, and everyone is encouraged to talk with one another about their experiences related to maintaining abstinence. Diversity and different opinions are respected, and there is an acceptance of each person's individuality and unique path into recovery. Although some may introduce themselves by acknowledging that they're an alcoholic or addict, this is not a requirement. Six guidelines are used to help people achieve their goal of abstinence.

Finding Out More

To learn more about this program and where meetings are held, SOS can be contacted at: SOS National Clearinghouse, The Center for Inquiry–West, 4773 Hollywood Blvd., Hollywood, CA 90026; tele-

phone: (323) 666-4295. They have two websites: www.cfiwest.org/
sos and www.secularsobriety.org, which contain all kinds of information about the program. Jim Christopher has written three books
about recovery without religion using the principles of SOS, and they
can be purchased through the SOS Clearinghouse.

SMART RECOVERY

SMART Recovery was developed in 1994 by a group of people who
were originally connected to Rational Recovery (RR). These people
decided to develop a separate program because RR altered its direction away from its original principles. SMART Recovery has maintained its allegiance to the original ideas of Rational Recovery.

The Program

SMART Recovery is the second largest self-help program for people
with alcohol problems (the largest being AA). SMART Recovery
doesn't view a problem with alcohol as a disease. It also does not
use the concepts of a "Higher Power" or powerlessness, nor does
it use the labels "alcoholic" or "addict." It does, however, maintain that abstinence must be the route to recovery. SMART Recovery is obviously very different from AA in terms of philosophy and
orientation.

SMART Recovery teaches self-reliance rather than reliance on a
Higher Power. It does not have sponsors. SMART Recovery under-
stands addiction as complex, learned, unhealthy behavior, or as a
complicated bad habit. Because SMART Recovery holds that people
have different needs and recover at different paces, it teaches that a
person's need to attend meetings will vary, and no one has to attend
meetings forever.

SMART Recovery uses scientific research and a "four-point pro-gram" in its meetings to help participants achieve abstinence. It helps individuals to (1) enhance and maintain their motivation to abstain from using alcohol or drugs, and (2) cope with urges and cravings to drink so that they don't have to act on them. Furthermore, people learn (3) rational ways to manage their thoughts, feelings, and be-haviors without using substances, and (4) to balance momentary and enduring satisfactions.

SMART Recovery also uses the "ABCs" to help people overcome their addiction, teaching that when something happens—an "**a**ctivat-ing event"—it leads to "**b**eliefs, thoughts, or attitudes," which can be irrational or illogical. These lead in turn to "**c**onsequences," which are emotions and behaviors. By better managing beliefs and emotions that lead to drinking, a person can empower himself to quit drinking.

Meetings are generally fairly small and are led by a "coordinator," who either is a person in recovery or someone who is knowledgeable about the program but who may never have had a drinking problem.

Finding Out More

SMART Recovery has more than three hundred groups both inside and outside the United States, and there are also many online meet-ings. You can contact them for meeting locations, recommended reading materials, and more information about the organization. Their address is: 7537 Mentor Avenue, Suite 306, Mentor, Ohio 44060; telephone: (440) 951-5357. Their website is www.smartrecov ery.org. Many books and publications about SMART Recovery can be found on their website. In particular, the *SMART Recovery Hand-book* offers a thorough overview of the program.

WOMEN FOR SOBRIETY

Women for Sobriety (WFS) was founded by Jean Kirkpatrick, Ph.D., in the mid-1970s. Dr. Kirkpatrick struggled with drinking, and after she found that AA no longer helped her, she began to stop drinking on her own by changing the way she thought about her problems. She came to believe that as a woman, she required specific treatment that focused on her self and self-confidence in addition to her alcohol problem. As she achieved success, she reached out to other women, which resulted in WFS.

The Program

WFS believes that heavy drinking is the way a woman learns to deal with emotional pain and that a part of recovery is learning healthier ways to deal with painful feelings and problems. WFS teaches its members to replace negative, destructive thoughts with positive, self-affirming ones. In addition, the strong message is given that all women are competent and can learn to be more self-reliant. In meetings, when a member introduces herself, she doesn't refer to herself as an "alcoholic," but rather as a "competent woman."

Meetings provide a place where women can talk with and receive support and encouragement from each other. WFS suggests that meetings remain small, six to 10 people, so that everyone can have the opportunity to talk and participate in the discussion that consists of a chosen topic related to drinking problems or something from WFS literature. Meetings are led by a member who has been abstinent at least one year and knows the philosophy of the WFS program. WFS also maintains a pen-pal program, so members can communicate by mail or email when not in meetings.

WFS uses the "New Life" Acceptance Program, which is based upon 13 statements (see p. 195). These statements offer suggestions for how members should deal with and think about life. WFS strongly encourages members to take control of their lives through thought and action. It also maintains that abstinence is the only route to recovery.

Finding Out More

For more information about WFS, contact WFS headquarters at: Women for Sobriety, Inc., PO Box 618, Quakertown, PA 18951-0618; telephone: (215) 536-8026. The WFS website, www.womenfor sobriety.org, contains a wealth of information about the program, including a listing of many publications and books that can be purchased. You can find out where meetings are held by calling WFS or by emailing them and telling them where you live. Two books to read in order to learn about WFS, both written by Jean Kirkpatrick, are *Turnabout: New Help for Women Alcoholics* and *Goodbye Hangovers, Hello Life: Self-help for Women.*

RATIONAL RECOVERY

Rational Recovery (RR) is included in this chapter because, at one point, RR was a self-help group. RR, however, changed its direction and is no longer a self-help group but a self-help resource. RR was started in the late 1980s by Jack Trimpey and used a type of therapy called Rational Emotive Therapy to help people with alcohol problems. Rational Emotive Therapy is an action-oriented therapy that teaches people to examine their own thoughts, beliefs, and behaviors and replace self-defeating ones with more productive alternatives. In the early 1990s, the focus of RR shifted to its present form.

THE "NEW LIFE" ACCEPTANCE PROGRAM

1. I have a life-threatening problem that once had me.
2. Negative thoughts destroy only myself.
3. Happiness is a habit that I will develop.
4. Problems bother me only to the degree that I permit them to.
5. I am what I think.
6. Life can be ordinary or it can be great.
7. Love can change the course of my world.
8. The fundamental object of life is emotional and spiritual growth.
9. The past is gone forever.
10. All love given returns.
11. Enthusiasm is my daily exercise.
12. I am a competent woman and have much to give life.
13. I am responsible for myself and for my actions.

© Women for Sobriety, Inc.

The Program

RR states that it is the antithesis and archrival of AA. RR avoids the beliefs of powerlessness and a "Higher Power." It also does not see an addiction to alcohol as a disease, nor does it believe that people need to be "in recovery" from their addiction to alcohol for the rest of their lives. RR maintains that people can completely "recover" and put their alcohol addiction behind them. The only thing RR and AA agree on is that abstinence is essential to control an alcohol problem.

When RR was originally developed, it held meetings and used the ideas of Rational Emotive Therapy. However, within a few years, RR shifted its philosophy and now uses AVRT, or Addictive Voice Recognition Technique. Furthermore, the leaders of RR began to believe that there was absolutely no need to go to meetings, and meetings were abolished. Thus, RR is not really a part of the self-help community. People achieve abstinence by visiting RR's website or by reading RR literature.

Using AVRT, people learn to disregard their "addictive voice"— the thoughts and feelings that support their addiction. Users of AVRT are taught to recognize and take control over their addictive voice. Recovery is an event, and abstinence can eventually become effortless.

Recently, RR has gone even further and now states that going to meetings or seeking any type of professional help is destructive to recovery because it takes away from personal responsibility. This thinking is incorporated into the organization's DPI, or Declaration of Personal Independence, which they encourage people to live by. The DPI states: "I will never, ever, attend another meeting of Alcoholics Anonymous or any other recovery group organization, nor will I obtain professional services of any kind, for the purpose of ending my addiction." RR believes that the way to beat an addiction is through traditional values of individual responsibility, resiliency, self-reliance, and personal independence. From my perspective, RR has taken things too far. While individual responsibility is important, there clearly is a place for professional treatment and self-help groups to assist people who struggle with their use of alcohol.

Finding Out More

You can find out more about RR by visiting their website at www
.rational.org. Their mailing address is: Rational Recovery Systems, Inc., PO Box 800, Lotus, CA 95651; telephone: (530) 621-2667; email: rr@rational.org. The book to read to learn more about RR is *Rational Recovery: The New Cure for Substance Addiction,* by Jack Trimpey.

16

PROFESSIONAL TREATMENT

Never give in! Never give in!
Never. Never. Never. Never.

WINSTON CHURCHILL

In addition to self-help groups, a whole system of professional care exists for you. Because different people require different types of care, a range of programs have been developed so that each person's specific needs can be met. Navigating this system can be confusing, as it's hard to know what kind of program you need, what kind of therapist to see, or even what's available. In this chapter, you'll learn about getting the care that's right for you.

You should know that the programs I review, in almost all cases, work for people with alcohol problems as well as those with drug problems or a combination of both alcohol and drugs. Therapists who specialize in the treatment of alcohol problems also generally specialize in the treatment of drug problems. I mention this because, if you get involved in any of these types of programs, you should expect that there may be some people there who struggle with drugs as opposed to alcohol. This, however, does not mean that these programs are not suitable for you. It is just that the professional treatment system is designed to work with people who struggle with substances, regardless of what the particular substance is.

INDIVIDUAL PSYCHOTHERAPY

Individual psychotherapy is a common choice for people who want help with their drinking. Some people prefer to speak to a therapist on a one-to-one basis instead of going to a self-help meeting. Others may wish to speak with a therapist in addition to attending some kind of self-help meeting, because they have some concerns they want to discuss privately with a trained professional. You may find that your mood does not improve even after staying sober and want to speak with someone to find out why you feel so bad. Psychotherapy can also be useful if you've been struggling to moderate your drinking and still want to see if you can learn to do so with some outside support.

Why Individual Therapy?

Individual therapy gives you the opportunity to look closely at yourself in a very private way. Within an individual psychotherapeutic relationship, you and your therapist can explore what has prevented you from resolving your alcohol problem and what you need to do to accomplish that goal. Together, you will identify stumbling blocks and ways to overcome them.

Individual therapy can also be particularly useful if, despite abstinence, you feel awful. Whether the painful feelings were always there and you used alcohol, at least in part, to cope with the feelings, or whether the feelings began after your drinking stopped, abstinence should not be a horrible, painful experience. Sure, some difficult times are to be expected. However, abstinence should not feel terrible, and therapy can often help you to understand your feelings and help you to move forward.

Choose the Right Therapist

When choosing a therapist, prior to making a first appointment, you should ask the therapist about his or her experience working with people who have alcohol problems. Don't be shy; this is critically important information. You should only see a therapist who has skill in working with problem drinkers. Even a very good therapist, if he or she is not specifically trained in the treatment of alcohol problems, will not provide you with the help you need. Your health insurance company will be able to give you the names of some therapists who specialize in this area. You can also look through the Yellow Pages or possibly get a referral through one of your friends or your primary care physician.

Many different kinds of professionals offer individual psychotherapy. The list includes alcohol counselors, social workers, marriage, family, and child therapists, psychologists, and psychiatrists. Often your insurance company will give you several names of therapists you can see. Choosing the right one is important, so how do you decide? If the only issue you are dealing with is your alcohol problem, it's fine to see any of these therapists, again, as long as they have the appropriate training in alcohol problems. However, if you have other concerns apart from your drinking problem, stick to ones who at least have a master's degree or higher (licensed clinical social workers, marriage, family, and child therapists, psychologists, and psychiatrists), because these people generally have additional training in issues other than alcohol. You should know, though, that psychiatrists often don't see people for therapy but only prescribe medications, so if you call a psychiatrist, inquire whether therapy is an option.

Whomever you see, within the first few sessions, you should feel that you can talk comfortably with your therapist and that this person can help you. In fact, if within the first or second session you feel that you can't talk with your therapist or that you just don't connect, you should shop around a little more to find a therapist with whom you feel comfortable.

There are also many, many different kinds of therapy. For example, behavior therapy places an emphasis on changing behavioral patterns that may cause you difficulties. In contrast, cognitive therapy focuses on identifying and correcting irrational and distorted beliefs that may be playing a role in your distress. And cognitive-behavioral therapy incorporates features of behavioral and cognitive therapy, focusing on both destructive behaviors and negative thoughts. Finally, psychodynamic therapy explores your past to better understand what prior events may be contributing to the beliefs, behaviors, and perception of the world that cause you problems. These are just four relatively common types of therapy; different therapeutic orientations number in the hundreds.

In my experience, therapists often incorporate features of many different approaches in order to best meet the needs of their clients. Thus, I wouldn't be particularly concerned with the type of therapy the therapist practices. Again, focus on how you feel you connect to your therapist after a couple of sessions and whether you feel this person can help you.

MARITAL AND FAMILY THERAPY

In marital and family therapy, you and other members of your family meet together with a counselor to resolve problems, conflicts, and tension between you and others. Even if you are already seeing a therapist individually, additional marital or family therapy may make sense if family problems are intense. In marital and family therapy, the focus isn't on you but rather on the relationships between family members. Sometimes even in individual therapy, one or more of your family members can be brought into the session to discuss a particular issue.

Whenever you plan to see a therapist for marital or family therapy, make sure that the person is skilled in this type of therapy. The nature of the work is very different than what occurs in individual therapy. Also make sure that the person knows about alcohol problems and how a family member's drinking can affect everyone within a family.

Why Marital or Family Therapy?

Drinking can cause a whole host of problems within your family, and even after you stop drinking, anger, resentment, mistrust, and other interpersonal problems can linger. People may not be talking to each other and tension may be high. Marital or family therapy can help to resolve those difficulties and get your family back on track.

GROUP THERAPY

Group therapy also can be helpful for the treatment of an alcohol problem. In groups you can learn from others what has and has not worked for them, and you can get honest feedback from peers. Moreover, you will discover that you're not alone, that others struggle with alcohol, and the support you can receive from the other members of the group can be invaluable. Certainly, the self-help group programs reviewed in the last chapter offer these same features, which, at least in part, explain their success. If you don't want to or don't feel comfortable attending a self-help group, but you still want a group experience, group therapy may be the answer. In general, most therapy groups will focus on abstinence from alcohol as the treatment goal, although there might be some exceptions.

Why a Group?

Group therapy, in contrast to individual therapy, offers the opportunity to share experiences with and to learn from others. If you think you would like this, as opposed to meeting with your own therapist, check out a group. I can't recommend individual therapy over group therapy or vice versa, as I think it depends upon your own personal preference. In contrast to self-help groups, in group therapy there will be a greater emphasis on personal problems you have and how these may be playing a role in your drinking. Helping you to work out particular concerns, to learn healthier ways to cope, and to improve difficult relationships are issues that can be addressed through group therapy.

Choose the Right Group

When considering group treatment, be sure that the focus of the group is to help people who have problems related to alcohol or drug abuse. A more general psychotherapy group will not focus on abstinence and learning how to accomplish this. If your goal is learning how to moderate your drinking, inform the group leader of this beforehand because a group with the goal of abstinence will not be suitable for you. You should also think about whether you prefer to be in a group with both sexes or one with only members of your own sex. Again, ask about this if it's important to you. Many outpatient treatment programs offer group therapy, and inquiries can be made about the availability of groups. Some private therapists also lead groups that might be appropriate for you.

INTENSIVE OUTPATIENT PROGRAMS

Intensive outpatient programs (IOPs) provide group treatment and support for people with an alcohol problem. These programs also offer individual therapy as well as educational and support meetings for family members. Most IOPs meet five or six days each week, from morning to mid- or late afternoon. Some programs meet for three hours each day; others meet for six. While the length of treatment is individualized, the program generally takes place over the course of one or two weeks, or possibly a little longer.

All IOPs offer a variety of psychoeducational and therapeutic groups, films, and discussions about aspects of substance abuse. Typical topics for group discussion generally include at least the following:

- the definition of an alcohol problem
- aspects of denial
- an alcohol problem as a family illness
- stress management
- dealing with urges
- leisure education and recreation
- coping with anger
- assertiveness training
- relapse warning signs and triggers

- relapse prevention
- an introduction to self-help groups
- coping with painful feelings

Some specialized groups, such as separate men's and women's groups, trauma groups, or groups for people who also have other psychiatric issues may also be offered.

The goals of the program are to educate you about the nature of alcohol problems and to teach the skills and coping mechanisms you need to achieve abstinence. You will learn about specific issues that may play a role in your inability to maintain abstinence and how to overcome your particular barriers to recovery.

Why an IOP?

An IOP is indicated for you if you've tried less intensive forms of treatment, such as self-help meetings or weekly individual or group therapy and haven't been able to achieve abstinence. These programs give you a lot of structure and can help you to develop a new lifestyle that doesn't include drinking. This type of treatment can help you build a basic foundation so that you can achieve and maintain abstinence.

If you haven't been able to achieve much success through other channels, an IOP can provide you with intensive treatment and the support you need. To find such a treatment program, look through the Yellow Pages under "Alcoholism" or "Alcohol Treatment" for a program in your area. If you have health insurance, your health insurance company will be able to provide you with such information, too. If you have been seeing an individual therapist and are continuing to struggle with maintaining abstinence, that person could also recommend an IOP. However, you need to be sure that your health insurance will pay for that particular program.

EVENING TREATMENT PROGRAMS

Evening treatment programs, created to accommodate work schedules, are similar to IOPs in that they offer a structured group therapy program to enable you to achieve abstinence. Generally, an evening treatment program meets three or four times a week over several weeks, although the actual length of stay varies based upon the amount of treatment you need to resolve your problem. As with IOPs, a variety of different groups and psychoeducational activities are provided.

Why Evening Treatment?

Of course, if you work during the day, an evening treatment program will be more convenient for you than a daytime program. Unlike most IOPs, evening treatment programs are more appropriate if you already have some ability to maintain abstinence, but you still occasionally relapse. While there are exceptions, evening treatment often offers less structure than an IOP. They may meet less frequently during the week and for a shorter period of time. In general, evening treatment is like fine tuning, whereas an IOP is akin to a basic-training program.

So if you have been able to put together some periods of abstinence, but still occasionally find yourself lapsing or relapsing, evening treatment should be considered. Evening treatment will focus closely on your relapse triggers, and relapse prevention is typically a major focus of treatment. You can find out about such a program by calling your health insurance company or by looking through the

Yellow Pages. When inquiring, be sure that the specifics of the program are appropriate for you.

RESIDENTIAL PROGRAMS

A residential program is any treatment program where you temporarily live. These include traditional inpatient detoxification programs, short-term rehabilitation programs, halfway house programs, and sober houses.

As was discussed in chapter 5, insurance companies generally have gotten away from paying for residential treatment except for inpatient detoxification, although there are some that still cover some limited residential care after detoxification. You may not require inpatient detoxification, but you may need to get involved in a structured residential treatment program away from your home environment if you haven't been able to achieve any long-term or significant periods of abstinence while living at home and utilizing outpatient treatment. So, if you are in this situation and your insurance does not cover this kind of treatment, what do you do?

Fortunately, there are various kinds of residential treatment options. Some programs are publicly funded, and others are private programs that people must pay for with their own resources. People are often referred to residential treatment after first being in an inpatient detoxification program. If you don't need detoxification but still need residential care, you can get involved in such a program if you can demonstrate that you're not currently using alcohol or other drugs. You can get information on specific programs in your area through your state department of public health, which will probably have an alcohol or substance abuse division that maintains a listing of all facilities. Other alcohol and drug abuse treatment programs will also have this information readily available.

Another great resource for finding a residential program, or any type of alcohol treatment program, is http://findtreatment.samhsa .gov, a website sponsored by the Substance Abuse and Mental Health Services Association (SAMHSA). This site lists all drug and alcohol facilities in the United States, and by clicking on the substance abuse treatment facility locator, you can find an appropriate program.

Rehabilitation Programs

Rehabilitation programs, or "rehabs," provide intensive education and structure in a residential setting. In such settings, groups, films, discussions, and AA or other self-help meetings are offered to build the skills you need to attain and maintain abstinence. One-to-one counseling is also available, which provides you with the opportunity to look closely at yourself and your alcohol problem. The time you spend in a residential program can vary from several weeks to a couple of months, or until an appropriate discharge plan has been developed. While some rehabs are coed, others may be only for men or only for women.

Why a Rehab? Rehabilitation programs can be helpful if you have been unable to benefit from other less structured forms of treatment and it is clear that you need a lot of education and skill building to attain abstinence. Rehabs will provide you with a temporary "time out" from your usual way of life and your usual friends, and they will give you the opportunity to work intensely upon yourself so that you can develop the skills needed to remain abstinent. These kinds of programs are appropriate if you have limited social support (e.g., sober family, partner, friends) to foster abstinence. If you have been unable to achieve abstinence, you should consider such a program.

Halfway Houses

Halfway houses are residential treatment programs that provide longer-term support. Many people enter a halfway house after first being in a rehab. The term *halfway* implies that the program is halfway between the community and the treatment world. Often, while living at the halfway house, you hold a job in the surrounding neighborhood, although some programs may restrict outside work. Halfway houses are usually supported by state funds and by their residents. Generally, residents pay rent to live at the program, just as anyone pays rent or a mortgage to live in an apartment or home.

Halfway houses differ in terms of their degree of structure. Some houses restrict privileges for several weeks after the person is first admitted to the program. For example, new residents may not be able to leave the grounds without a staff member or a longer-term resident of the program, and obtaining an outside job may not be allowed or may be put off for a period of time. Others immediately or fairly quickly allow and encourage residents to resume employment. How much free time is provided also varies between programs, as does the amount of treatment offered. Some have frequent in-house meetings and require residents to attend AA or other self-help meetings in the community. Others offer and require less formal treatment.

How long you live in a halfway house also varies and is based upon your need for continued treatment and on the structure of the program. In general, the time period may be for several months to one year. When contacting a halfway house for possible admission, ask about the rules and requirements of the program to ensure that you are entering the type of program you want.

As with rehabs, some halfway houses are coed, but others may be just for men or just for women. There are also some specialized halfway houses, although they are not as numerous. For example, some are only for adolescents, others are primarily for gay individuals, and others are designed for women who want to live there with their children.

Why a Halfway House? Halfway houses are needed if you have a serious alcohol problem and require intensive and long-term treatment to stay sober. These programs also offer a living environment that is alcohol-free, and this can be particularly helpful if you don't have a living arrangement that can support your abstinent lifestyle. Because all residents in the halfway house are attempting to achieve abstinence, you can get considerable peer support. The feeling that "we are all in this together, trying to get our lives together by not drinking" can be quite powerful, and it helps to counter the notion that you are struggling all alone against the world.

You should consider this type of program if you repeatedly have been unable to achieve abstinence in the community and if people in your home drink significantly. After you leave a short-term rehab, a halfway house may help you build the foundation for long-term abstinence.

Sober Houses

Sober houses are similar to halfway houses in that a group of individuals who are all trying to achieve abstinence live together in a home, providing support to one another. However, they offer less structure and treatment than halfway houses.

Sober houses are often used as a "step-down" after an individual completes a halfway house program. Individuals also can enter them directly from the community or from an inpatient detoxification or rehabilitation program. Some sober houses offer little, if any, formalized treatment or structure, whereas others have some limited ongoing groups and supports, so be sure to inquire about this. Sober houses are supported by the residents who pay rent to live there.

Why a Sober House? Like halfway houses, a sober house can provide a support system to help you to get back on your feet and achieve long-term abstinence. You should consider such a program if you have been unable to maintain abstinence on your own, your home situation is not supportive of a non-drinking lifestyle, and you feel that you could benefit from living with others who are also trying not to drink.

17

MEDICATIONS

The brain is the most complex object of human inquiry.

JAMES H. BILLINGTON, D.Phil., Librarian of Congress,
and STEVEN E. HYMAN, M.D., Director,
National Institute of Mental Health

During the last 20 years or so, there has been an explosion in our knowledge of the brain. Technologies have been developed that help us better understand how this complex organ works, including some ideas about how alcohol interacts with the brain, what it is about alcohol that makes people want to drink it, and why alcohol can be hard to quit. As a result, some new medications have been produced specifically for the treatment of an alcohol problem.

There are currently three types of medication available to help people with a drinking problem stop drinking:

- Antabuse (disulfiram)
- ReVia (naltrexone)
- Campral (acamprosate)

Disulfiram has been around a long time, but naltrexone and acamprosate are much newer. These medications work in very different
ways, and all must be prescribed by a physician.

As alcohol problems are very complex and these medications work
in such different ways, there has been some research that has studied
whether taking two of these drugs together may have an even greater
benefit. In general, the results of this research have been mixed—
some studies have shown this to be beneficial, but others have not.
More studies are needed and it is possible that, for some people, this
could be helpful. You can speak with your doctor about whether a
combination of these medications might be indicated for you.

Before I discuss each of these medications, the most important
thing you need to know is that they are all *tools* to help you stop
drinking. None is a *total treatment program.* If you are still struggling
to stay sober, don't think that simply taking a medication will turn
everything around for you. In our society there is the belief that most
any problem can be solved with a pill or a capsule. You have a cold?
Take a drug. A headache? Take a drug. A backache? A drug. You want
to lose weight? Take a drug. Feeling stressed? Here's a drug. And the
list goes on and on. Although the medications mentioned here can be
extremely helpful, it takes more than medication alone to overcome
an alcohol problem. As you've learned, recovery is a lifestyle change
and medication cannot, nor is it designed to, do that.

DISULFIRAM (ANTABUSE)

Disulfiram is a drug that discourages you from drinking. If you take
disulfiram and drink, you'll become quite ill. Symptoms you can
experience include: flushing of the skin; a throbbing headache; nausea or even vomiting; sweating; anxiety; chest pain; palpitations; and

hyperventilation and respiratory distress. An extreme reaction can bring on shock and cardiac arrhythmia.

How It Works

When alcohol is consumed, it is broken down to *acetaldehyde* by an enzyme called *alcohol dehydrogenase*. Acetaldehyde is then converted to acetic acid by *acetaldehyde dehydrogenase*. Disulfiram blocks acetaldehyde dehydrogenase, causing acetaldehyde to build up in the blood system. Acetaldehyde is very toxic and causes the alcohol-disulfiram reaction I just described.

If you take disulfiram, the fear of experiencing a painful reaction to alcohol stops you from drinking. If you take disulfiram every day, you don't even need to seriously think about drinking because you know, beyond a doubt, that if you drink you will get very, very sick.

Of course, the protection against drinking that disulfiram provides works only if you take it. If you aren't motivated to stop drinking, you'll find a way not to. Maybe you'll "forget" to take it. And, inevitably, at some point in the not-too-distant future, you'll start to drink again. In fact, on some level you probably stopped taking it because you made the decision to drink again.

You must be highly motivated to stop drinking if you're going to continue to take disulfiram, because you know that mixing the two will get you very sick. You should be aware that a reaction to disulfiram can occur up to 14 days after the last dose is taken.

Things to Know

Because disulfiram reacts highly to alcohol, you need to be careful to avoid all types of alcohol. For example, you should not eat pastry or candy that contains alcohol. In fact, you shouldn't do this anyway because, regardless of where alcohol comes from, if you are abstaining from alcohol, it needs to be avoided—period. You don't want to eat or drink any alcohol, since even a very small amount can slowly escalate to your ingesting more and more, as reviewed in chapters 10 and 13. You also need to avoid products like mouthwash, cough syrups, or other medications that contain alcohol. There is also a small risk of having a disulfiram reaction to aftershave lotions and perfumes that contain alcohol, so you need to read labels carefully. Your doctor can review with you the things that you need to avoid.

On the other hand, if you eat food in which alcohol has been used in the cooking process, the alcohol has usually evaporated, so this should not be a problem. Pastries with vanilla extract, for example, should not be problem. If excessive amounts of alcohol have been used, however, like wine in some sauces, some alcohol can remain, which could cause a reaction. In general, it is best to be more rather than less cautious.

As with all medications, there can be some side effects to disulfiram, most of which are generally mild. In addition, not everyone can take disulfiram for medical reasons. Only your physician can make the decision whether disulfiram is suitable for you. If you are interested in trying disulfiram, speak with your physician, who can answer your specific questions. If you are very motivated to stop drinking, this medication, along with all of the other things you can do to help yourself, should be considered.

NALTREXONE (REVIA)

Naltrexone is a much newer agent than disulfiram and works in a significantly different way. Rather than making you sick if you drink alcohol, it can help to take away a craving for alcohol. If you do drink, you won't experience the same feelings of intoxication that you used to, so it may help to stop you from experiencing a major relapse, as you won't want to drink more and more.

How It Works

Endorphins are naturally occurring opioids that we all have in our bodies. Opioids are painkillers, and these natural opioids cause euphoria, sedation, and a sense of well-being when they attach to certain areas in the brain called receptor sites.

When you drink, endorphins are released and attach to the receptor sites in your brain that cause the pleasurable feelings you get by drinking. One idea to help a person who struggles with an alcohol problem is to prevent endorphins from attaching to those receptor sites. If this is done, alcohol will no longer have the same effect, so the person won't want to drink as much. Naltrexone does just this. If you drink and are taking naltrexone, you won't feel the usual euphoria, pleasure, and well-being. As you no longer get the same "kick" from drinking, you won't want to drink, or at least you won't want to drink as much.

Research has found that people who took naltrexone reported less overall drinking than people who did not take naltrexone, and when they drank, a major relapse occurred less often. Interestingly enough, people who took naltrexone also reported significantly less craving for alcohol than people who were not taking it. Exactly how naltrexone decreases craving is not entirely clear, but it appears to have this effect. So if you struggle with intense cravings and urges to drink, I strongly recommend that you give naltrexone a try.

There is also an injectable form of naltrexone called Vivitrol that works in the same exact way. Vivitrol lasts for an entire month, and you can see your doctor, who can give you a shot. The advantage of taking naltrexone this way is that you don't have to remember to take it every day but only have to remember to see your doctor on a monthly basis. This is a good alternative for you if you don't like to take a daily pill or don't think that you will remember to take it every day.

Things to Know

As with all medications, naltrexone can have some side effects, but these are generally mild. There are also some individuals who should not take naltrexone due to their medical conditions. In particular, if you have significant liver disease or elevated liver enzymes, you can't take naltrexone. If you are interested in trying this medication, make an appointment with your physician to see if it's right for you.

You should also know that because naltrexone blocks all opioids from attaching to those receptor sites, it will prevent other opioid-type drugs from acting in the body. What this means is that if you need an opioid-type painkiller for an injury or other reason, it won't work. Other methods of combating pain will need to be used instead. Your doctor can discuss this with you and suggest other pain medications that you can take.

ACAMPROSATE (CAMPRAL)

Acamprosate is the newest medication used to treat people with alcohol problems. Like naltrexone, acamprosate helps to reduce the cravings you can experience when you first stop drinking. As a result, acamprosate is best prescribed right after you stop using alcohol. It is recommended that acamprosate be taken for at least one year. So if you experience strong cravings to use, especially right after you first stop drinking, you should consider acamprosate.

How It Works

It is not entirely clear how acamprosate works, but it has something to do with restoring the imbalance of chemicals (*neurotransmitters*) in your brain that can be caused by heavy drinking. A number of studies conducted in Europe and the United States have shown that rates of abstinence were greater among people who took acamprosate than among people who took a placebo. In addition, the total number of days of not drinking was also higher among the people who took acamprosate.

Things to Know

As with disulfiram and naltrexone, acamprosate needs to be prescribed by a physician, and there are some people who can't take this medication for medical reasons. For example, some individuals can be hypersensitive to this drug and experience an allergic reaction to it. Those with severe renal impairment cannot take it either. Your physician can determine whether this drug is indicated for you.

PSYCHIATRIC MEDICATIONS

In chapter 16, I mentioned that some people who stop drinking continue to feel bad, and I suggested individual or group psychotherapy. There are times, though, when therapy alone may not help. Psychiatric medication may be needed to treat specific symptoms that may be completely separate from a person's alcohol problem.

It is quite common for problem drinkers to have other psychiatric problems. In fact, a study conducted by the National Institute of Mental Health found that among people who have ever experienced an alcohol problem, a little over one-third had experienced a psychiatric disorder at some point in their lives. Common psychiatric problems were depression, anxiety, and bipolar disorder, which is a mood disorder characterized by feelings of extreme highs and lows. In fact, the chance of someone with an alcohol problem having a psychiatric disorder is about double that of people who have never had an alcohol problem.

Fortunately, many medications target neurochemical processes in our brains that relate to psychiatric complaints. A psychiatrist is able to determine whether a particular medication should be taken for a specific psychological difficulty, although other mental health professionals such as psychologists and social workers often have a pretty good sense of when medication may be needed. Such individuals make referrals to psychiatrists who will determine whether medication makes sense and what type of medication should be prescribed.

Who Doesn't Need Medication

Many people who stop drinking may suffer from some emotional distress but don't need and should not be prescribed medication. Their solution involves learning new ways to cope that don't include alcohol. For example, at the time you decide to do something about your drinking problem, you may feel miserable, awful, and down. You may also be anxious about the current problems in your life, many of which may have been caused by your drinking. This is further compounded by the fact that you must now deal with these problems without alcohol, your usual way of coping.

So, initially, you may feel troubled and overwhelmed when you first stop drinking. Your solution, though, is learning how to manage your problems without drinking, either on your own or with the support of therapy. As you do this, you'll find that, pretty quickly, you start to feel better with no need for medication.

Who Needs Medication

For some people, medication is an essential treatment intervention if they are ever going to feel better. For example, without medication, people with bipolar disorder will continue to experience intense mood swings that will make their lives unmanageable. Without stabilizing their moods, it can be difficult or impossible for them to abstain from alcohol. Such people *need* medication as a component of their overall recovery program.

While bipolar disorder is a serious psychiatric condition, others experience more subtle difficulties that also require medication. You may have resolved your drinking problem and made the necessary changes to support your new life, yet you may continue to feel mildly or severely depressed. I have seen many people who report feelings of depression and can't pinpoint why they continue to feel so miserable. Often, they report that things in their lives are good and that, despite having no reason to feel bad, they do. Medication can help to resolve those feelings so they can enjoy life again. Other people may experience considerable difficulty getting a handle on their drinking problem due, in part, to their depression. Medication has often played an important role in enabling these people to finally resolve their drinking problem. So if you have stopped drinking and are working hard to make the lifestyle changes that go along with it, but you continue to feel bad, medication should be considered.

Most importantly, don't think that nothing can be done, or that it's your fault that you continue to feel bad, or that you are doing something wrong. Your individual effort may have nothing to do with it, and you should proactively make an appointment to see a psychiatrist, who can make the final determination whether some type of medication makes sense for you.

For some of you, this may be a big step. It may be hard to admit you need this help, or you may view it as a "crutch." But try not to see it this way. Instead, accept that certain people need appropriate medication to feel better. It's just that simple. For many psychiatric disorders, medication is the treatment of choice, just as insulin is for the treatment of diabetes, or as antibiotics are for the treatment of an infection. A psychiatrist who is knowledgeable about alcohol problems can help to determine whether medication might benefit you.

When to Start Medication

Professionals working in the field used to think that a person who had a drinking problem should not be prescribed psychiatric medication for at least six months to one year after they resolved their drinking problem. This stemmed from the belief that a person could not be diagnosed with an emotional disorder until alcohol had been out of their system for this period of time. This, however, is no longer believed, and medication can be prescribed even shortly after a person first stops drinking. If you need medication, but it isn't started, it will decrease the chance that you'll be able to stop drinking. Or even if you are able to stop, you will continue to feel bad.

On the other hand, it is impossible to know if you need medication if your drinking remains out of control. Alcohol is a powerful drug and can affect how you feel. For example, if you feel depressed, your drinking may be responsible for these feelings, or at least contributing to them. So while medication can be started early on, a period of abstinence is needed to make a proper diagnosis and decision about whether medication should be prescribed. So even if you feel bad and think that drinking helps you to cope, you owe it to yourself to take a break from drinking so that you can be properly evaluated.

Things to Know

If you see a psychiatrist for a medication evaluation, be sure to tell her that you have struggled with alcohol consumption, because certain medications should not be prescribed to you. Some medications have the potential to be abused, particularly by people who have a history of excessive alcohol or drug use. Your psychiatrist will also review with you the potential problems of drinking while taking any prescribed medication.

If you are prescribed medication for a psychiatric problem, this doesn't mean that your alcohol problem is no longer important or doesn't still need your focus and attention. Your psychiatric problem, while it may have played a role in the development of your alcohol problem and may continue to have an influence on it, is not entirely responsible for your alcohol problem. Both problems exist, and you must address both of them.

Even when your psychiatric problem is properly treated and you're feeling better, your alcohol problem doesn't go away. You still have a vulnerability to drink too much, and you need to focus on this.

AFTERWORD

*Always bear in mind that your own resolution to
succeed is more important than any one thing.*

ABRAHAM LINCOLN

In this book, I hope I have helped you to understand what an alcohol problem is and how to take control of your problem so that you can help yourself. By using the techniques offered here, you may discover that you are able to help yourself and require no outside treatment. On the other hand, if you have difficulty helping yourself, I have also outlined the available treatments.

There is no one type of treatment that is appropriate for everyone. Everyone is different, and these differences must be respected. Whether you help yourself on your own or want or need some outside help is not important. Neither is how you choose to understand your drinking problem or whether you address your alcohol problem through abstinence or are able to learn moderation. What is important is that you have taken control of your problem and are finally doing something about it.

Some final words of advice:

- Be honest with yourself. If you want a better life, you must acknowledge your problem with alcohol.
- Never lose sight of your commitment to change.
- Remember the painful, troublesome consequences of your drinking. These problems are the reasons you have decided to address your drinking. Remembering them will help you to stay focused on your decision. Focus will help you to succeed.
- Work hard to create a fulfilling life for yourself without alcohol. Life can be very enjoyable, even without drinking.
- If you cannot consistently moderate your drinking, you need to accept this, move on, and work to achieve abstinence.
- Despite wanting to drink, you can still choose not to drink. Urges to drink go away even without drinking.
- It may take time to begin to feel better, but you will if you stay with it. Remember that returning to drinking is not the answer and will only make you feel worse in the long run.
- Never give up on yourself. You are worth the effort.
- Learn from your mistakes.
- Never stop trying. You are the only one who can get the job done.

> *You can do what you want to do, accomplish what you want to accomplish, attain any reasonable objective you may have in mind—not all of a sudden, perhaps not in one swift and sweeping act of achievement—but you can do it gradually, day by day and play by play, if you want to do it, if you work to do it, over a sufficiently long period of time.*
>
> WILLIAM E. HOLLER

NOTES

INTRODUCTION

xiii   Rate of alcohol problems among adults in the United States:
Grant, B. F., Dawson, D. A., Stinson, F. S., Chou, S. P., Dufour,
M. C., and Pickering, R. P. 2004. The 12-month prevalence
and trends in DSM-IV alcohol abuse and dependence: United
States, 1991–1992 and 2001–2002. *Drug and Alcohol Dependence*
74: 223–34.

xv   About 75% of people who struggle with alcohol resolve their
drinking problem on their own and without treatment:
Sobell, L. C., Cunningham, J. A., and Sobell, M. B. 1995. Recovery
from alcohol problems with and without treatment: Prevalence
in two population surveys. *American Journal of Public Health*
86: 966–72.

CHAPTER 1. DO YOU HAVE A DRINKING PROBLEM?

9–11   Seltzer, M. L. 1971. The Michigan Alcoholism Screening Test: The
quest for a new diagnostic instrument. *American Journal of Psychiatry* 127: 89–94.

CHAPTER 2. WHY DOES DRINKING CAUSE YOU DIFFICULTY?

16   Sigmund Freud wrote several papers on his observation that people often get stuck in a certain way of being in the world and that,
despite suffering from this, they continue to repeat the same thing
over and over. See:
Freud, S. 1920/1961. *Beyond the Pleasure Principle* (J. Strachey, ed.
and trans.). New York: Norton.

17–18   "Disease," *Webster's Ninth New Collegiate Dictionary.* 1993. Spring-
field, MA: Merriam-Webster.

19–20   Alcohol problems as a disease:

American Society of Addiction Medicine. 1990. *ASAM News* March-April.

Jellinek, E. M. 1960. *The Disease Concept of Alcoholism.* New Haven, CT: Hillhouse Press.

Rush, B. 1810. *Medical Inquiries and Observations upon the Diseases of the Mind.* New York: Hafner.

Woodward, S.B. 1838. *Essays on Asylums for Inebriates.* Worcester.

20–23   Genetic vulnerability to develop an alcohol problem:

Goodwin, G. W. 1979. Alcoholism and heredity. *Archives of General Psychiatry* 36: 57–61.

Heath, A. C., Madden, P. A., Bucholz, K. K., Dinwiddie, S. H., Slutske, W. S., Bierut, L. J., Rohrbaugh, J. W., Statham, D. J., Dunne, M. P., Whitfield, J. B., and Martin, N. G. 1999. Genetic differences in alcohol sensitivity and the inheritance of alcoholism risk. *Psychological Medicine* 34: 451–53.

National Institute on Alcohol Abuse and Alcoholism. 1992. The genetics of alcoholism. *Alcohol Alert* no. 18 PH 357.

Schuckit, M. A. 1985. Ethanol-induced changes in body sway in men at high alcoholism risk. *Archives of General Psychiatry* 43: 375–79.

Schuckit, M. A. 1988. Reactions to alcohol in sons of alcoholics and controls. *Alcoholism: Clinical and Experimental Research* 12: 465–70.

Schuckit, M. A., and Smith, T. L. 2000. The relationships of a family history of alcohol dependence, a low level of response to alcohol and six domains of life functioning to the development of alcohol use disorders. *Journal of Studies on Alcohol* 61: 827–35.

Schuckit, M. A., Goodwin, D. W., and Winokur, G. 1972. A half-sibling study of alcoholism. *American Journal of Psychiatry* 128: 1132–36.

Vaillant, G. E. 1983. *The Natural History of Alcoholism.* Cambridge, MA: Harvard University Press.

26–27   Documentation that people with alcohol problems can learn to moderate their drinking:

Armor, D. J., Polich, J. M., and Stambul, H. B. 1978. *Alcoholism and Treatment.* New York: John Wiley and Sons.

Davies, D. L. 1962. Normal drinking in recovered alcohol addicts. *Quarterly Journal of Studies on Alcohol* 23: 94–104.

Kendell, R. E. 1965. Normal drinking by former alcohol addicts. *Journal of Studies on Alcohol* 44: 68–83.

Vaillant, G. E. 1983. *The Natural History of Alcoholism.* Cambridge, MA: Harvard University Press.

27–28 People with drinking problems can be taught to drink less and control their drinking:

Miller, W. R., and Hester, R. K. 1980. Treating the problem drinker: Toward an informed eclecticism. In *The Addictive Behaviors: Treatment of Alcoholism, Drug Abuse, Smoking, and Obesity,* ed. W. R. Miller. Elmsford, NY: Pergamon.

Miller, W. R., and Hester, R. K. 1989. Treating alcohol problems: Toward an informed eclecticism. In *Handbook of Alcoholism Treatment Approaches,* ed. R. K. Hester and W. R. Miller. Elmsford, NY: Pergamon.

Sobell, M. B., and Sobell, L. C. 1973. Alcoholics treated by individualized behavior therapy: One year treatment outcome. *Behavior Therapy and Research* 11: 599–618.

Sobell, M. B., and Sobell, L. C. 1976. Second year treatment outcome of alcoholics treated by individualized behavior therapy. *Behavioral Research Therapy* 14: 195–215.

CHAPTER 3. GETTING READY AND STAYING MOTIVATED

44 Learned helplessness experiment:

Seligman, M. E. P., Mater, S. F., and Geer, J. H. 1968. Alleviation of learned helplessness in the dog. *Journal of Abnormal Psychology* 73: 256–62.

CHAPTER 4. CAN YOU REALLY HELP YOURSELF?

49 The quotation from Robert Dupont comes from the following:

Dupont, R. L. 1983. Foreword. In *Treating Adolescent Substance Abuse,* by G. R. Ross. Boston: Allyn and Bacon.

49–50 Many people who struggle with their drinking are able to help themselves without treatment:

American Psychiatric Association. 1994. *Diagnostic and Statistical Manual of Mental Disorders,* fourth edition. Washington, DC: American Psychiatric Association Press.

Institute of Medicine. 1990. *Broadening the base of treatment for alcohol problems.* Washington, DC: National Academy Press.

50–51   People resolving their problem with alcohol without treatment:

Dawson, D. A. 1996. Correlates of past-year status among treated and untreated persons with former alcohol dependence: United States, 1992. *Alcoholism: Clinical and Experimental Research* 20: 771–79.

Sobell, L. C., Cunningham, J. A., and Sobell, M. B. 1995. Recovery from alcohol problems with and without treatment: Prevalence in two population surveys. *American Journal of Public Health* 86: 966–72.

Vaillant, G. E. 1983. *The Natural History of Alcoholism.* Cambridge, MA: Harvard University Press.

54   The individual is the key ingredient in behavior change:

Hubble, M. A., Duncan, B. L., and Miller, S. D. 1999. *The Heart and Soul of Change.* Washington, DC: The American Psychological Association.

CHAPTER 5. YOU MAY NEED MEDICAL HELP

63   People who had an extended stay in a hospital did no better than those who had a much shorter stay and got involved in outpatient treatment:

Fink, E. B., Longabaugh, R., McCrady, B. M., Stout, R. L., Beattie, M., Ruggieri-Authelet, A., and McNeil, D. 1985. Effectiveness of alcoholism treatment in partial versus inpatient settings: Twenty-four month outcomes. *Addictive Behaviors* 10: 235–48.

CHAPTER 6. WHAT TO DO: ABSTINENCE OR MODERATION?

66–70   Rates of successful controlled drinking and the type of drinker who has the best chance to learn to control drinking:

Dawson, D. A. 1996. Correlates of past-year status among treated and untreated persons with former alcohol dependence: United States, 1992. *Alcoholism: Clinical and Experimental Research* 20: 771–79.

Sobell, L. C., Cunningham, J. A., and Sobell, M. B. 1995. Recovery from alcohol problems with and without treatment: Prevalence in two population surveys. *American Journal of Public Health* 86: 966–72.

Vaillant, G. E. 1983. *The Natural History of Alcoholism.* Cambridge, MA: Harvard University Press.

CHAPTER 8. YOUR PERSONAL MODERATE DRINKING CONTRACT

86   On limits for low-risk drinking:

Dawson, D. A., Grant, B. F., and Li, T. K. 2005. Quantifying the risks associated with exceeding recommended drinking limits. *Alcoholism: Clinical and Experimental Research* 29: 902–8.

National Institute on Alcohol Abuse and Alcoholism. *Alcohol Alert* no. 16 PH 315, April 1992.

World Health Organization, Department of Mental Health and Substance Dependence. 2000. *International Guide for Monitoring Alcohol Consumption and Related Harm.* Geneva: World Health Organization.

CHAPTER 10. MANAGING YOUR THOUGHTS TO QUIT DRINKING

127   Forty-eight percent of adults living in the United States do not drink:

National Institute on Alcohol Abuse and Alcoholism. http://pubs .niaaa.nih.gov / publications / Practitioner / CliniciansGuide2005/ guide.pdf

CHAPTER 11. WHAT YOU MUST DO TO QUIT DRINKING

143   Aerobic exercise and meditation may have a positive benefit on overall mood:

Infante, J. R., et al. 1998. ACTH and beta-endorphin in Transcendental Meditation. *Physiology and Behavior* 64: 311–15.

Yeung, R. 1996. The acute effects of exercise on mood state. *Journal of Psychosomatic Research* 40: 123–41.

CHAPTER 12. MANAGING URGES TO USE

151   On nutritional deficiencies associated with heavy drinking:

National Institute on Alcohol Abuse and Alcoholism. *Alcohol Alert* no. 22 PH 346, October 1993.

CHAPTER 13. SLIPS AND FALLS ON THE PATH TO SOBRIETY

164   The most common reasons for relapse:
Levy, M. 2001. Building a system to prevent relapse. *Behavioral Health Tomorrow* 10: 34–37.

CHAPTER 15. SELF-HELP GROUPS

186   AA publications:
Alcoholics Anonymous. 1952/1976. *Alcoholics Anonymous.* New York: Alcoholics Anonymous World Services, Inc.
Alcoholics Anonymous. 1952/1981. *Twelve Steps and Twelve Traditions.* New York: The AA Grapevine and Alcoholics Anonymous World Services, Inc.

189   Information on MM:
Kishline, A. 1994. *Moderate Drinking: The Moderation Management Guide for People Who Want to Reduce Their Drinking.* New York: Crown Trade Paperbacks.

191   On SOS:
Christopher, J. 1988. *How to Stay Sober: Recovery without Religion.* Amherst, NY: Prometheus Books.
Christopher, J. 1989. *Unhooked: Staying Sober and Drug Free.* Amherst, NY: Prometheus Books.
Christopher, J. 1992. *SOS Sobriety: The Proven Alternative to 12-Step Programs.* Amherst, NY: Prometheus Books.

192   On SMART Recovery:
SMART Recovery Handbook. Available through the SMART Recovery online bookstore, www.smartrecovery.org.

194   On Women For Sobriety:
Kirkpatrick, J. 1986. *Goodbye Hangovers, Hello Life: Self-help for Women.* New York: Atheneum.
Kirkpatrick, J. 1990. *Turnabout: New Help for Women Alcoholics.* New York: Bantam.

196   On Rational Recovery:

Ellis, A., and Grieger, R. 1986. *Handbook of Rational-Emotive Therapy*, vol. 2. New York: Springer.

Trimpey, J. 1996. *Rational Recovery: The New Cure for Substance Addiction.* New York: Pocket Books.

CHAPTER 17. MEDICATIONS

212   For research on combination of medications:

Anton, R. F., O'Malley, S. S., Ciraulo, D. A., Cisler, R. A., Couper, D., Donovan, D. M., Gastfriend, D. R., Hosking, J. D., Johnson, B. A., LoCastro, J. S., Longabaugh, R., Mason, B. J., Mattson, M. E., Miller, W. R., Pettinati, H. M., Randall, C. L., Swift, R., Weiss, R. D., Williams, L. D., and Zweben, A. 2006. Combined pharmacotherapies and behavioral interventions for alcohol dependence: The COMBINE study: A randomized controlled trial. *Journal of the American Medical Association* 295: 2003–17.

Besson, J., Aeby, F., Kasas, A., Lehert, P., and Potgieter, A. 1998. Combined efficacy of acamprosate and disulfiram in the treatment of alcoholism: A controlled study. *Alcoholism: Clinical and Experimental Research* 22: 573–79.

Petrakis, I. L., Polig, P., Levinson, C., Nich, C., Carroll, K., and Rounsaville, B. 2005. Naltrexone and disulfiram in patients with alcohol dependence and comorbid psychiatric disorders. *Biological Psychiatry* 57: 1128–37.

215   On naltrexone:

O'Malley, S. S., Jaffe, A. J., Chang, G., Schottenfeld, R. S., Meyer, R. E., and Rounsaville, B. 1992. Naltrexone and coping skills therapy for alcohol dependence. *Archives of General Psychiatry* 49: 881–87.

Volpicelli, J. R., Alterman, A. I., Hayashida, M., and O'Brien, C. P. 1992. Naltrexone in the treatment of alcohol dependence. *Archives of General Psychiatry* 49: 876–80.

Volpicelli, J. R., Clay, K. L., Watson, N. T., and Volpicelli, L. A. 1995. Naltrexone and the treatment of alcohol dependence. *Alcohol Health & Research World* 18: 272–78.

217   Benefits of acamprosate:

Mann, K., Lehert, P., and Morgan, M. Y. 2004. The efficacy of acamprosate in the maintenance of abstinence in alcohol-dependent individuals: Results of a meta-analysis. *Alcoholism: Clinical and Experimental Research* 28: 51–63.

217–18 More than one-third of people who experience an alcohol problem may suffer from some type of psychiatric illness:

Regier, D. A., Farmer, M. E., Rae, M. S., Locke, B. Z., Keith, S. J., Judd, L. L., and Goodwin, F. K. 1990. Comorbidity of mental disorders with alcohol and other drug abuse: Results from the Epidemiologic Catchment Area (ECA) Study. *Journal of the American Medical Association* 264: 2511–18.

INDEX

social factors (*continued*)
88–89, 92–95, 99; of moderation vio-
lations, 110–15; of seeking treatment,
48–50, 56–57
social support system, 54, 56; for abstinence, 146–47, 171; community programs, 63, 208–10; limited, 207–10;
for managing urges, 157–58; for moderation, 93, 96–98, 104. *See also* self-
help groups
social worker, 176, 199–200, 218
special populations, 203–4, 209
sponsors, in self-help groups, 184, 191
statistics on alcohol abuse, xiii
"step-down" programs, 210
stigma, problem drinking as, viii–ix, 3,
14–15, 29
stress, 17, 82–83, 93, 153, 162, 221
stress management. *See* relaxation
Substance Abuse and Mental Health
Services Association (SAMHSA),
207
substance abuse treatment programs,
64; intensive outpatient, 203–5
success with moderation: honesty and,
108–16; personal conditions for, 65,
69–70, 161
support. *See* social support system
support groups, therapeutic outpatient,
203–4. *See also* self-help groups
surveys on self-help vs. treatment, 50–
51

taste, focus on, 78, 88
therapeutic support groups, 203–4
thinking the drink through, 155–57,
164–65
thirst, 78–79

thoughts: for confronting denial, 166–
69; daily, for abstinence, 127–30, 134;
irrational, 80, 192, 194, 200; managing for quitting, 125–37; for managing urges, 154–57, 164–65
time: alcohol-free, 140–41; as healer,
133, 170
time of day, drinking and, 91
time period for quitting, 129–32
treatment: as essential, 49–52; long-
term benefits, 56–57, 68; medications, 211–24; personal choices, vii–
xiv, xvi, 223; professional, 154, 171,
197–210; research review, 27, 50–51;
seeking outside, 175–78; self-help
groups vs., 179–96; self-help vs., 49–
52, 56–57; where to begin, xv–xvi,
176
trial period: of abstinence, 43; of moderation, 71–72
triggers: of lapses/relapses, 161–66, 169,
171; of urges, 130, 152–53, 165–66
Twelve Steps of AA, 182–83

urges to use: feelings and, 153–54; managing, 149–52, 154, 158; moderation
and, 83; passing without drinking,
154–57; supportive efforts for, 157–
58; triggers, 130, 152–53, 165–66

vitamin deficiencies, 151
Vivitrol (naltrexone), 215–16

wanting to drink, 151, 164–65
weakness perspective, personal, 13, 15–
17, 177
web sites, 171, 186, 189–91, 196, 207
weight, drink limits and, 87